HASHISH:
Studies of Long-Term Use

Hashish:
Studies of Long-Term Use

Editors

Costas Stefanis, M.D.

Professor and Chairman
Department of Psychiatry
University of Athens School of Medicine
and
Chief of Psychiatry
Eginition Hospital
Athens, Greece

Rhea Dornbush, Ph.D.

Senior Research Scientist
Reproductive Biology Research
  Foundation
St. Louis, Missouri

Max Fink, M.D.

Professor of Psychiatry
State University of New York
  at Stony Brook
Stony Brook, New York
and
Executive Director
International Association for
  Psychiatric Research, Inc.
Great Neck, New York

Raven Press ■ New York

Raven Press, 1140 Avenue of the Americas, New York, New York 10036

Made in the United States of America

Library of Congress Cataloging in Publication Data
Main entry under title:

Hashish: studies of long-term use

    Bibliography: p. 159
    Includes index.
    1. Hashish--Psychological aspects. 2. Hashish--
Physiological effect. I. Stefanis, Costas.
II. Dornbush, Rhea L. III. Fink, Max. [DNLM:
1. Cannabis. 2. Drug dependence--Occurrence--Greece.
WM276 H348]
BF209.C3H37   615'.782   76-19848
ISBN 0-89004-138-5

Foreword

This volume represents an important link in a chain of publications resulting from a series of studies on the health consequences of chronic cannabis use that was sponsored by the United States National Institute on Drug Abuse (NIDA). In the wake of public anxiety about the epidemic increase of marijuana use in the late 1960s, the predecessor of NIDA, the Center for Studies on Narcotic and Drug Abuse, then part of the National Institute of Mental Health, had initiated three studies in foreign countries where cannabis use is more traditional and/or has a longer history than in the United States. The first study was of ganja use in Jamaica, followed by the one on hashish users in Greece, and, most recently, marijuana use in Costa Rica. Each has had a slightly different work scope as the questions raised about the drug have grown increasingly complex and sophisticated.

Since the use of cannabis is embedded within the social and cultural matrix of the respective countries, it should be kept in mind that many of the effects and the interpretation of those effects are biased by expectation, set and setting, and it takes sophisticated statistical methodology to extract meaningfully generalizable conclusions. The present authors make a successful attempt to explore and indicate the nature of this social matrix in Greece. Beyond that, they have also been successful in demonstrating some important pharmacological consequences of hashish: the acute effects on physiological and psychological processes and the clear existence of pharmacological tolerance to Δ-9-THC in chronic hashish users.

The conclusions presented in this volume with regard to the long-term health consequences of cannabis are largely reassuring. Hashish, a relatively potent form of cannabis, was not found to produce brain damage, at least as evidenced by sophisticated techniques of electroencephalography, echoencephalography, and psychological testing. The authors found no evidence of either an organic mental syndrome or of an amotivational syndrome in their working-class subjects. The users, however, did exhibit a higher incidence of psychopathology, although it was unclear whether or not it was related to hashish use. The medical findings generally were indistinguishable from those in the control population.

While these findings indicate that marijuana is not the feared "killer weed" that previous well-meaning but emotionally biased reports would have us believe, this report does not give hashish or marijuana a clean bill of health. The present volume may appear to be too technical to some readers; nevertheless, it provides just the kind of scientific data that is necessary to make us better informed as to the true nature of this drug. The conclusions that are drawn are carefully qualified by the authors. They realize that "the principal limitation of the present studies of long-term users in Greece, Jamaica, and Costa Rica is the small sample size in each study." They feel that they may be studying the healthy and resistant survivors of the drug habit and may have missed the possible victims who are not available. This is a general problem with this type of retrospective study that can be eliminated only by longitudinal prospective types of studies.

Prospective studies are costly, lengthy, and, by necessity, have to focus on a few, well-defined questions on large subject populations. To be able to launch such a large-scale prospective study, we have to sort out the meaningful questions from the peripheral ones obtained in well-controlled retrospective studies and take the basic, preclinical data into consideration for possible clues. We at NIDA are presently engaged in accumulating this type of data and the present volume, together with the Jamaican and the soon to be published Costa Rican data, will serve as important data bases for this process. This lengthy, painstaking data gathering and evaluating process, we feel, is necessary to generate valid, scientific information to dispel popular myths about marijuana and hashish. Ultimately this will help to elevate the quality of discussions and of the decision-making process regarding the status of cannabis in society to a more rational level.

S. Szara
*National Institute
on Drug Abuse,
Washington, D.C.
January 7, 1977*

Preface

During the 1960s national and international unrest accompanied the continuing cold war between Eastern Europe and the West. In the United States protests against the conscription of young men in an escalating undeclared war in Indo-China led to campus upheavals, street strife, and the tragedies at Kent State University. An important aspect of the confrontations between the national leaders and the youth of America was a demand for "law and order"—a euphemism for the illegal and quasilegal exercise of police power to coerce American youth into conformity, not only in regard to military conscription but also in their dress, hair styles, and drug use.

One manifestation of the hostility between the state and its citizens was the preoccupation with drug abuse by governmental agencies and the communication media. By the middle of the decade, concerns about opiate abuse were prominently voiced in the press; and by 1967–68 interest was focused on cannabis abuse. Campus "busts" of marijuana users became front-page news, and reports of the dangers of cannabis use appeared with increasing frequency in the public and scientific press.

During the spring of 1968 Dr. C. J. Miras, Professor of Biological Chemistry at the University of Athens, presented his observations of personality disorders among long-term hashish users and his typology of the chronic hashish user at a number of scientific meetings in the United States. His data included electroencephalographic (EEG) records from subjects who had used hashish for more than two decades. These records were filled with extensive slow-wave activity, which, if they were representative of alert subjects in an otherwise nontoxic state, could be viewed as evidence for chronic brain damage.[1,2] Dr. Miras encouraged detailed studies of these subjects, and later that year Dr. Henry Brill of the New York State Narcotic Addiction Control Commission visited Dr. Miras in Athens and confirmed the clinical state of these subjects.

In May 1969, during a visit to Athens, I examined them with Professor Miras. The subjects (men) reported using hashish for 10–30 years, with recent smoking of five to six water pipefuls daily. They said they maintained their jobs, homes, and family lives. They described symptoms of irritability, anxiety, and unpredictable outbursts when they failed to obtain hashish each day, and said they were relaxed and drowsy after each smoking of hashish. During these examinations there was no evidence of an organic mental syndrome or chronic deterioration in their affect, response to questions, or motor behavior.

During that visit, the electrophysiology laboratories of Professor Costas Stefanis were found to be fully equipped for the studies of the chronic hashish users suggested in the discussions with Professor Miras. Professor Miras exhibited a wide range of cannabis substances, as well as growing facilities at the university, which assured us of an adequate supply of active material. With the cooperation of Drs. Miras and Stefanis, we proposed to examine the feasibility of detailed studies of the effects of long-term hashish use.[3]

The feasibility study, undertaken during the summer of 1971, demonstrated that a population of cooperative long-term heavy hashish users was available for extensive neurophysiological and psychological testing.

During the subsequent 3 years, this population was examined in a variety of studies. The first defined the social, medical, neurological, and psychological characteristics of the user population, and compared these with a carefully matched nonuser population. We also assessed how representative the user population was in relation to the known national hashish user population in Greece. A second study assessed the acute effects of smoking cannabis substances in chronic users. The physiological, psychological, and behavioral effects of the inhalation of various cannabis substances were defined. A third study examined the effects of withdrawal of hashish in these long-term users.

Concurrently, the staff at the New York Medical College was examining the effects of smoking cannabis substances in young, American occasional users. The same methods and substances were used for many of the evaluations in Athens. The projects in New York provided a testing ground for the methods used in the Athens populations.[4]

During the assessment of these populations we were aware of the ongoing studies in Jamaica and, later, as we completed our studies, the onset of the studies in Costa Rica. The data of the Greek studies were not presented publicly while the study was in progress in the belief that careful assessment of the total study would provide the best evaluation of the findings.[5]

In the context of the heightened interest in cannabis in the 1960s, this volume represents a major effort of scientists to answer the questions of concern to the public. We are aware that the issues surrounding cannabis legislation and proscription are primarily political. Nevertheless, these scientific studies were done to determine the facts in nature, in the hope that their clarification will relieve the anxiety of some citizens whose children or family members may have become involved with cannabis.

Max Fink

---

[1]Miras, C. J. (1971): Marihuana and hashish. Presented in a lecture at the University of California at Los Angeles.

[2]Miras, C. J. (1972): Studies on the effects of chronic cannabis administration to man. In: *Cannabis and Its Derivatives*, edited by W. D. M. Paton and J. Crown. Oxford University Press, London.

[3]This proposal was funded by the United States National Institute of Mental Health on June 22, 1970 (HSM 42-70-98) through the International Association for Psychiatric Research, Inc.

[4]These studies were supported by the National Institute of Mental Health through the New York Medical College (MH 18172).

[5]The material reported here was presented in part at the Pharmacology of Marijuana meeting in December 1974. Published in: Dornbush, R., and Kokkevi, A. (1976): The acute effects of various cannabis substances on cognitive, perceptual, and motor performance in very long-term hashish users. In: *Pharmacology of Marihuana*, edited by M. C. Braude and S. Szara, pp. 383–391. Raven Press, New York, and Fink, M., Volavka, J., Panayiotopoulos, C. P., and Stefanis, C. (1976): Quantitative EEG Studies of marijuana, delta-9-tetrahydrocannabinol, and hashish in man. In: *The Pharmacology of Marihuana*, edited by M. C. Braude and S. Szara, pp. 383–391. Raven Press, New York. ; at the meeting of the American Psychiatric Association in May 1975 Published in: Stefanis, C., Liakos, A., Boulougouris, J., Fink, M., and Freedman, A. M. (1976): Chronic hashish use and mental disorder. Am. J. Psychiatry, 133:225–227. ; and at the New York Academy of Sciences Conference on Chronic Cannabis Use, held under the auspices of the New York Medical College, the National Institute of Drug Abuse, and the New York Academy of Sciences in January 1976. Published in: Dornbush, R. L., Freedman, A. M., and Fink, M. (1976): Chronic Cannabis Use. Annals NY Acad Sci, 282.

Acknowledgments

This study was made possible by the support, cooperation, and encouragement of many collaborators. We are deeply indebted to Professor Alfred M. Freedman of the New York Medical College for his encouragement and advice; to Dr. Henry Brill of the New York State Department of Mental Hygiene and the National Commission on Marihuana and Drug Abuse for recommending this study be undertaken; and to Professor C. Miras of the University of Athens for directing so many of the subjects to us, for the supplies and the assays of cannabis substances, and for a willingness to look at data that differed from his initial findings. Financial support was obtained from the Grants and Contracts Management Branch of the U.S. National Institute of Mental Health (now National Institute on Drug Abuse) under contract HSM 42-70-98. Drs. Steven Szara, Robert Petersen, and Monique Braude were particularly encouraging. Additional support was obtained from the International Association for Psychiatric Research, Inc., Great Neck, N. Y. (Mr. T. J. Israel, Jr., President, 1970–1974). The New York Medical College studies were supported in part by NIMH grant MH 18172.

We are grateful to Mrs. V. Liakos and Mr. Bassiakos of Athens, and Mr. P. Irwin of New York, for their technical assistance in the electrophysiological studies.

For the successful conclusion of this project, the senior investigators are indebted to the many fellow scientists and agencies cited above and to co-workers and friends throughout the world who freely shared their techniques and experiences with us.

Contents

Foreword vii

1. Sociocultural Aspects of Hashish Use in Greece 1
    Costas Stefanis, Costas Ballas, and Demitra Madianou

Sample Selection and Methods

2. Selection and Definition of Users and Controls 11
    *Aris Liakos, Demitra Madianou, Costas Ballas, and Costas
    Stefanis*

3. Methods of Acute Inhalation Experiments 21
    *Rhea Dornbush, John Boulougouris, Jan Volavka, and Anna
    Kokkevi*

4. Methods of Withdrawal Study 25
    Rhea Dornbush, Aris Liakos, and Anna Kokkevi

Results: Sample Characteristics

5. Characteristics of Hashish Users and Controls: Social, Family, and Personal 33
    *John Boulougouris, Aris Liakos, Demitra Madianou, and
    Costas Stefanis*

6. Subjective Experiences of Cannabis Use in Long-Term Users   39
    John Boulougouris and Aris Liakos

7. Psychological Test Characteristics of Long-Term Hashish
    Users 43
    Anna Kokkevi and Rhea Dornbush

8. Incidence of Mental Illness in Hashish Users and Controls .. 49
    Costas Stefanis, John Boulougouris, and Aris Liakos

9. Medical Studies in Long-Term Hashish Users. I. Physical and
    Neurological Examinations 55
    John Boulougouris, E. Antypas, and C. P. Panayiotopoulos

    Medical Studies in Long-Term Hashish Users. II. Clinical
    Electroencephalography and Echoencephalography 59
    *C. P. Panayiotopoulos, Jan Volavka, Max Fink, and Costas
    Stefanis*

Results: Acute Experiments

10. Acute Subjective Experiences on Inhaling Different Cannabis
     Substances 63
     John Boulougouris and Rhea Dornbush

11. Acute Effects of Cannabis on Cognitive, Perceptual, and Motor
     Performance in Chronic Hashish Users 69
     Rhea Dornbush and Anna Kokkevi

12. Acute EEG Effects of Cannabis Preparations in Long-Term
     Hashish Users 79
     Jan Volavka, Max Fink, and C. P. Panayiotopoulos

13. Visual Evoked Responses in Chronic Hashish Users 91
     C. P. Panayiotopoulos and Costas Stefanis

14. Intercorrelations Between Physiological and Psychological Ef-
     fects of Marijuana, Hashish, and THC-Δ-9 in Long-Term
     Hashish Users 95
     Peter Crown, Rhea Dornbush, and Jan Volavka

15. Psychophysiological Effects of Acute Cannabis Inhalation ... 103
     Aris Liakos, John Boulougouris, and Costas Stefanis

Results: Withdrawal Studies

16. Ad Libitum Consumption and Abstinence 111
     Rhea Dornbush and Max Fink

17. Withdrawal from Cannabis: Psychological Test Performance   121
     Rhea Dornbush and Anna Kokkevi

18. Withdrawal from Cannabis: Psychophysiological Changes ... 135
     *John Boulougouris, Aris Liakos, Costas Stefanis, Rhea
     Dornbush, and C. P. Panayiotopoulos*

19. Withdrawal from Cannabis: Laboratory Tests and Clinical Ob-
     servations 147
     *Costas Ballas, John Boulougouris, Aris Liakos, and Costas
     Stefanis*

20. Study of Long-Term Hashish Users in Greece: Summary and
     Discussion 151
     Max Fink

     References 159

     Index ..../.................................... 171

Contributors

Costas Ballas, M. D.
Department of Psychiatry, University of Athens School of Medicine; and Eginition Hospital, Athens, Greece

John Boulougouris, M.D.
Department of Psychiatry, University of Athens School of Medicine; and Eginition Hospital, Athens, Greece

Peter Crown, Ph.D.
Department of Psychiatry, New York Medical College, New York, New York 10029

Rhea Dornbush, Ph.D.
Reproductive Biology Research Foundation, St. Louis, Missouri

Max Fink, M.D.
Department of Psychiatry, State University of New York at Stony Brook, Stony Brook, New York 11790; and International Association for Psychiatric Research, Inc., Great Neck, New York

Anna Kokkevi, M.A.
Department of Psychiatry, University of Athens School of Medicine; and Eginition Hospital, Athens, Greece

Aris Liakos, M.D., Ph.D.
Department of Psychiatry, University of Athens School of Medicine; and Eginition Hospital, Athens, Greece

Demitra Madianou, M.A.
Department of Psychiatry, University of Athens School of Medicine; and Eginition Hospital, Athens, Greece

C. P. Panayiotopoulos, M.D., Ph.D.
Department of Psychiatry, University of Athens School of Medicine; and Eginition Hospital, Athens, Greece

Costas Stefanis, M.D.
Department of Psychiatry, University of Athens School of Medicine; and Eginition Hospital, Athens, Greece

Jan Volavka, M.D., Ph.D.
Missouri Institute of Psychiatry, St. Louis, Missouri 63139

1

Sociocultural Aspects of Hashish Use in Greece

Costas Stefanis, Costas Ballas, and Demitra Madianou

To put the present study of long-term hashish users in Greece in perspective, it is useful to present the principal historical and cultural reasons why Greeks did not incorporate hashish smoking into their cultural inventory until the middle of the nineteenth century, and to define the reasons which led to its adoption by only one part of the Greek population, a section best considered as a cultural subgroup (175a).

CANNABIS IN EUROPE

The available facts convince us that cannabis moved rapidly from the highlands of central Asia to the European mainland. Reininger (158) describes cannabis seeds and hulls among remnants of herbs in a pot of the third century BC found in a tomb near Wilmersdorf, Germany. These are the only known relics from antiquity. No reference to cannabis is made in either the Egyptian papyri or the New Testament.

The first reference to the use of cannabis in Europe appears in Herodotus (IV, 74–75) about 450 BC. He mentions that the Scyths not only cultivated cannabis and used it as a euphoriant, "they threw cannabis seeds on red-hot stones and became drunk by inhaling the smoke." It seems certain that the Scyths, as mentioned by Papadopoulos (141), were using not only the seeds, which are devoid of euphoriant properties, but also the tufts of the female plant. Herodotus reports that cannabis grew wild in Thrace, but that it was cultivated for its fibers, which were used for weaving.

Cannabis was used widely in western Europe for commercial purposes during the pre-Roman period. Athenaeus (AD 170–230) reports that the tyrant of Syracuse, Hieron II, who lived between 270 and 215 BC, obtained cannabis from the valley of the Rhone in order to manufacture rope for his navy. Pliny the Elder (AD 23–79) notes that the sails and canvas of the Roman galleys were made from cannabis fiber.

It has not yet been established how cannabis reached Europe from Asia. It may have arrived through Russia to northern Europe or from the Middle East through the Mediterranean ports and the Aenos peninsula to southeastern Europe. Both routes are probable. The possibility should not be overlooked, however, that cannabis may have been cultivated in northern Europe at the same time it was in Asia, a view supported by Hartwich (74). Nevertheless, the etymology of the word cannabis favors the view that the Middle East was the main avenue of cannabis traffic from Asia to Europe. The word cannabis is probably derived from the Assyrian words *qunubu* and *qunabu,* which signify "a way to produce smoke."

CANNABIS AND ANCIENT GREECE

We lack evidence that cannabis was used by the early Greeks for commercial, ritual, or euphoriant purposes. Herodotus, the Greek historian, mentions that "some other people" (the Scyths) were using cannabis. There is no reference suggesting that *nectar,* the "sweetdrink" of the Olympian gods, contained cannabis, as did *soma,* the favorite drink of the God Indra, which was offered to mortals so they might find happiness. We also lack evidence that cannabis was used at the Aesculapian shrines or at the Oracles. The plants principally used at these sites to modify consciousness were the solanaceae, hyoscyanus albus, datura stramonium, and mandragora. The prophetic delirium of Pythia has been ascribed to the inhalation of cannabis, but there is no evidence to corroborate this hypothesis (8).

Cannabis may have been used in ancient Greece, but no mention is made of it in the principal sources which would be likely to refer to it. Theophrastus (372–287 BC), a master of the peripatetic school, described the plants known to grow in Greece in great detail but makes no mention of cannabis. Plutarch (AD 46–127), however, in his work *On Rivers and Mountains' Names* (1615) mentions (400 years after Herodotus) that the people of Thrace used a herb similar to oregano, the tops of which they threw into the fire after meals and, inhaling their smoke, became drunk and fell into deep sleep.

Cannabis is described by Dioscorides (AD 59–79), a Greek doctor of the Roman army whose *Materia Medica* remained a standard for centuries. Dioscorides wrote that cannabis has two varieties, wild and domestic. The domestic variety produced a tall plant; the stems were used for making strong rope, and the seeds were used pharmaceutically. He recommended the seeds for curbing sexual desire and the fluid extract for earaches. Papadopoulos (141) doubts the plant that Dioscorides described as "wild" to be cannabis, since Dioscorides mentioned that it had red flowers.

Galen (AD 131–201), the Greek physician of Pergamum, emphasized the euphoriant qualities of cannabis. He observed that abuse or overdose of cannabis caused sterility (Galen 1821–33; Vol. XII) and that "the seeds produce stomach trouble, headache, and a disturbance of the body 'humours.' However, some people use them with other 'tragimata,' beverages that are taken after dinner to produce pleasure" (Galen 1821–33; Vol. V).

Cannabis is also mentioned by Pausanias, the geographer and traveler who lived during the second century. In his *Description of Greece*, he refers to cannabis but does not indicate whether it was used by the Greeks during the Roman period. His citation that "The land of Elis is fruitful, being especially suited to the growth of fine flax. Now while hemp and flax, both the ordinary and the fine variety, are sown by those whose soil is suited to grow it, the threads from which the Seres make the dresses are not produced from bark, but in a different way" is misquoted by Reininger (158) when he claims that Pausanias mentions that cannabis was cultivated in Elis in northwestern Peloponnesus.

BYZANTINE EMPIRE

The Byzantine Empire constituted a state combining Hellenic culture, Greek language, Christian religious beliefs, and Roman political traditions. Within its boundaries, it encompassed several ethnic groups: Greeks, Latins, Syrians, Armenians, Mesopotamians, and even North Africans. It has been categorized primarily as an Orthodox-Christian state and only secondly as a Greek state.

The Greek inhabitants of Byzantium came into contact with Moslem Arabs centuries before its conquest by the Turks. By the seventh century the Arabs had captured many provinces, including Alexandria and Jerusalem. Crete and Cyprus were recaptured by the Byzantines only after lengthy wars. The close geographical and social contact of Arabs and Byzantines enabled the former to become familiar with the Greek language and culture. Arabs gradually adopted Greek as an international language of communication with other nations.

The Moslem Turks replaced the Arabs in occupying the outer rim of the Byzantine provinces. By 1250 they had expanded their domination to a much larger part of the Byzantine Empire and also adopted Greek as their diplomatic language. For example, Mehmet II, the conqueror of Constantinople, spoke Greek eloquently. The influence of Hellenism on the Moslem world was matched by the Moslem influence on Byzantine cultural patterns. There is no evidence, however, to indicate that Byzantine Greeks, conquered first by Arabs and then by Turks, acquired the use of narcotics, either opium or hashish.

Thus we have no evidence that cannabis was used by the Greeks either during the classical era or the Roman period. During these times cannabis was an exotic plant used by the non-Greek peoples of Thrace and Scythia. This conclusion may also be extended to the Greeks of the Byzantine period; and it appears certain that cannabis, in contrast to alcohol, was not important in the cultural life of Byzantium.

OTTOMAN OCCUPATION

The fall of Constantinople in 1453 was followed by the dissolution of Byzantium. Within two centuries the occupation of the entire Greek peninsula, with the exception of the Ionian Islands, was complete. Many Greeks escaped to western countries, and many were lost during the persecutions and slaughters that followed each new conquest, especially that of Constantinople. A large part of the Greek population, however, survived and remained under Ottoman rule.

The survival of a Greek subculture was due largely to the policies of Mehmet II after 1453. He granted substantial religious and administrative privileges to Christians and allowed the organization of an autonomous community life. These policies may have been dictated by the need to secure financial support from Christian subjects, primarily for maintenance of the army.

Tolerance toward Christian subjects, which persisted for four centuries, allowed the Greeks to organize themselves into legal communities and to enjoy freedom of movement and worship. They were thus able to preserve their customs, religious and educational institutions, and even their national and cultural identity.

The available sources (144) indicate that the Christian population, and particularly the Greeks, did not assimilate into Moslem society. The literature of the Turkish occupation does not refer to the use of hashish by Greeks, so we must assume that the basic euphoriant for the Greeks continued to be alcohol.

Hashish smoking was common among the Moslems of the Ottoman Empire. Its use was more prevalent among the Moslem inhabitants of Arabic origin than among Turks. A painting in Nicolas de Nicolay's book, reproduced by Stringaris (179), depicts a group of Turkish soldiers in the streets of Constantinople, around 1500, inebriated by hashish. An epic poem, the "Benk u Bode," written by the Turkish poet Mohammed Ebn Soleiman Foruli of Bagdad in the middle of the sixteenth century, deals allegorically with a dialectical battle between wine and hashish (65). Under the guise of a fencing match, the poem describes with surprising accuracy the euphoriant properties and the consequences of the use of the substances. Foruli's poetry ranks the two substances on the basis of social criteria. This was also emphasized by Brunel (23), considering wine the drink of the rich and powerful (he likens it to a Sheikh, a guest of the Sultan), "while hashish is the friend of the poor, the Dervishes and the men of knowledge, i.e., of all those who are not blessed with earthly goods and social power." This description indicates that the Turks, at least those of higher social status, by the sixteenth century had already begun to adopt the habits of the conquered population and were indulging in alcohol, despite Koranic prohibition.

The distribution of hashish, alcohol, and opium use among the population of occupied Constantinople was reported by Eulogio Efendi, the Turkish historian of the seventeenth century (179). He describes the existence of more than 1,000 beer shops, 104 wine distributors, and only 60 "tekes" (hashish smoking places). The view that hashish was disseminated mainly by Dervish sects (a Dervish religious school even existed in Athens under

Turkish rule, and its building may still be seen in Monastiraki) and among the poor Turks is supported by other sources. Kerim (100) mentions that hashish was widely known in Syria, Asia Minor, Constantinople, Prusa, and in the environs of Smyrna. In each of these communities the Greeks lived symbiotically with the Turks.

GREECE AFTER THE LIBERATION

The modern Greek state was founded in 1830 after a war of independence, with only one geographic area then inhabited by Greeks included. In total area it encompassed 47,516 km² with a population of 753,000. In 1870, with the annexation of the Ionian Islands, the Greek land mass increased to 50,221 km² and the population to 1,457,000. By 1920, with the annexation of Macedonia, Epirus (in 1912), and West Thrace, Greece expanded to 127,000 km² with a population of 5,016,889. After the arrival of the displaced Greeks from Turkish Asia Minor in 1922, the population had increased in 1928 to 6,204,684; and with the annexation of the Dodecanesus in 1947, its geographic expanse had enlarged to the present 131,944 km². The population of Greece in 1971 was recorded as 8,768,641. In this 10-fold increase in population and tripling of its physical size within 150 years, many Greeks from diverse subcultures were brought within the polity, acquiring a greater homogeneity in language, religion, and national identity (167). The economic base of the nation, at least to the end of the last century, was predominantly agricultural. It is significant that in 1853 there were only three cities with a population of over 10,000: Hermoupolis, capital of the island of Syros; Athens; and Patras, the port of western Peloponnesus (190).

Hashish was not traditionally used as a folk medicine in Greece. Dionysos Pyrros, a Thessalian who studied medicine in Italy and had a vast knowledge of folk remedies, does not mention hashish in his *Doctor's Handbook*, printed in 1832 (152). "Cannabis semen-Cannabis sativa" is mentioned in the first official Greek *Pharmacopoeia* issued in 1837: "a yearly plant, indigenous in the East but also growing in Europe when planted." Cannabis is also mentioned by the first professor of pharmacology at the University of Athens, N. Kostis, in his 1855 *Handbook of Pharmacology*: "a plant, indigenous in the East and especially in Persia, but cultivated in many areas of Europe and Greece." He classifies this plant in his section on "Pharmaca Mucilaginosa" but not in the narcotics category. Cannabis is first mentioned as a narcotic in 1875 by Th. Afendoulis in his *Pharmacology*, described as follows: "Herrba siva Summitates foribuendae Cannabis indicae, a plant, indigenous in India and cultivated there as well as in Egypt, recently also in Greece in the areas of Argolis and Navpaktos in the Peloponnesus. In medicine as well as in everyday life, flowering tops of the female plant are used by Indian, Egyptian, and Arab peoples." This author also refers to the use of cannabis derivatives by Easterners and Egyptians in the diet.

Many sources refer to hashish as definitely appearing in Greece after 1850.

Introduced from the East, its starting point was the island of Syros in the Cyclades (110,141,179). An analysis of the demographic, social, and cultural status of this island, therefore, is of considerable interest.

Until 1790 the population of Syros was 4,000, with the majority Catholic (as a result of the Venetian occupation) and Greek-speaking. Following the war of independence in 1821 and the Turkish persecution of the inhabitants of other Aegean islands (Chios, Psara, Crete, Rhodes), many fled to Syros. These refugees established the town of Hermoupolis about the harbor, while the older Catholic inhabitants remained in Ano Hora, the old village in the hills above the new town. The growth of Hermoupolis was rapid, for it shortly became the leading port of the nation—so much so that English businessmen identified Syros as Greece. These changes occurred when many wealthy Greeks were living outside Greece in Constantinople, Austria, Rumania, or Russia.

An urban-commercial society with the first beginnings of industry was formed in Hermoupolis. By 1828 it was the largest city of Greece, with a population of 14,167 drawn from various parts of the nation. The majority were from Chios and other islands of the Aegean, later followed by Greeks from Asia Minor; the new inhabitants concentrated on new commercial enterprises and related industry. Hermoupolis quickly became an important port of call, a necessary stopover between East and West, between North Asia and the Black Sea. Until 1880 it maintained its national leadership in commerce and industry; the first Greek shipyards and factories were established in Hermoupolis. As a result, this city developed the first urban proletariat of Greece and the first labor syndicates; and it experienced the first strikes and labor unrest as well. As social counterpoint to this laboring class, a strong bourgeoisie emerged and flourished. In its social activities, life style, and habits this latter group closely resembled the western European bourgeoisie.

The older Catholic stratum of Syros was initially contained in the area known as the Kastro, in the hills above the city. These Catholic Greeks retained a traditional style of life based on agriculture and were culturally alienated from the urban life of the port city. Nevertheless, beginning in 1890, given the growing demands of new enterprises, these agricultural people began to be drawn into the urban labor pool. In spite of the antipathy between the Catholic inhabitants of Kastro and the rich Greek Orthodox newcomers of the port (numerous clashes have been recorded), the Catholics were eventually forced to seek work as longshoremen and ship-yard hands, and in the tanning factories of Hermoupolis, coming to the port to work by day and returning to their village by night—the first Greek example of migration for urban work without physical abandonment of the village. Although the needs of the port and of the flourishing factories and commerce lured workers from all of Greece, the first true proleteriat was recruited from Kastro.

These workers developed a distinctive social form with a characteristic cultural style. Syros became the meeting place of eastern (primarily Arabian) and western European influences. In Hermoupolis laborers were exposed to both as ships and crews from Europe, Egypt, and the Middle East made it a regular port of call. Among other elements of culture, Syros was introduced to western European music, which was quickly adopted by the upper class, and was applied to Arabic and Middle Eastern musical forms (192). As important, however, the refugees from the Peloponnesus, mainland Greece, and Pontos brought the tradition of Greek demotic songs.

The blending of these elements created a variant type of folk culture, tangentially related to that of the middle class but clearly differentiated. Within this multicultural context, a music form developed with overt oriental characteristics and influence; the basic instruments were the *bouzouki* and the *baglamas,* which bear resemblance to the mandolin and guitar. This new music developed in Syros but was soon transplanted to Piraeus, the seaport of Athens, from there to be spread to working people in all the harbors of mainland Greece. After World War II this music acquired significant dimensions and diffused rapidly throughout the Greek lower class. From 1950 on it could be considered the national music of the country. Popularly known as *rebitiko* music, it is socially akin to American blues and jazz (192).

Because of economic developments in continental Greece, from 1870 Piraeus began to compete commercially with Syros. By 1880 it had gained ascendancy, and with the opening of the Corinth Canal in 1893 the decline of Hermoupolis commenced. At this point the labor force gravitated away from Syros toward Athens and Piraeus. We maintain that the roots of hashish use in Greece are to be found in the Syros type of sociocultural setting. During the cultural flowering of this island, similar social, economic, and cultural events took place in Smyrna, an important port city of Turkish Asia Minor with a basically Greek population which dominated local trade and industry. In view of close similarities between the development of Smyrna and Syros, the use of hashish by the inhabitants of Smyrna cannot be dismissed. This view is strongly supported by reports that many of the Asia Minor Greeks repatriated in 1922 were hashish users.

The first reports of hashish smoking on the mainland occur around 1870–1880, at a time when socioeconomic conditions in Piraeus were comparable to those experienced by Syros (110, 179). One report mentions that hashish was introduced by the prisoners of Smyrna, Mysiri, and Prusa as the "weed of the poor" (148). It was the poor of Piraeus and its surrounding neighborhoods that constituted the bulk of the hashish-smoking population of the region.

It is probable that the cultivation of hashish was introduced to Greece around 1875 by immigrants from Egypt, Cyprus, and other eastern areas. By the last decade of the nineteenth century, hashish was openly cultivated for local use and export (178). Papadopoulos (141) estimates that before 1915 approximately 26,000 acres in Greece were put to hashish cultivation.

From the onset and until the 1960s, hashish use in Greece was limited to the working class, being widely used by longshoremen, boatmen, sailors, porters, skinners, slaughterers, cart drivers, and later truckdrivers (179). The spread of hashish use is correlated with the development and dissemination of *rebetiko* music (148). As hashish use became an element in the behavior and personality of *rebetiko* musicians and singers, the development of this musical genre and the proliferation of its practitioners became intimately linked to the dynamics of the hashish cult (179).

Stringaris (179) reports that the first admissions in 1885 to a newly established mental hospital, Dromokaiteion, were hashish users, diagnosed as mentally disturbed. Our own review of the hospital's files finds the first admissions of mentally disturbed hashish users to have been in 1912, with admissions of morphine and cocaine addicts recorded as starting in 1901. Until 1937 the prevailing term for institutionalization due to hashish use was "hashish mania;" after that date, the term is replaced by "hashish psychosis." Even until 1941 there were some admissions utilizing this terminology. From 1943 to 1947 hashish users admitted to Dromokaiteion were diagnosed as having "mixed or other toxicomanias."

On March 27, 1890, following a decision of the Medical Council, the Greek Department of Interior issued a circular prohibiting the importation, cultivation, and use of hashish as an imminent threat to society (178). Despite passage of this restrictive law, in force until 1920, hashish was regularly used in the *tekedes* (cafes frequented by hashish smokers), in the harbor area of Piraeus, and in the center of Athens. The habitues of *tekedes* were mostly young, jobless, tough men who as a rule subsisted by illegal activities and were usually at odds with the law and the authorities. Known quite widely in Greece as *manges*, they had their own code of honor and a paradoxically tender and touchy personality; they fiercely rejected the established social order (148).

Hashish use flourished during the decade following the first World War. Greek soldiers, returning home after the war in Asia Minor, brought back hashish smoking habits they had learned in Turkey (38); and approximately 1.5 million Greek refugees from the destroyed areas of Asia Minor were repatriated to Greece. Among this population were individuals who either smoked or knew about hashish. It is probable that the poor living conditions to which they were subjected after repatriation in the slum areas of Tavros, Assyrmatos, Kokkinia, and Drapetsona contributed to an increase of hashish smoking and to the establishment of more *tekedes*. The problem is more complex, however. The population that came from Asia Minor consisted primarily of war widows and children in need of immediate relief and support which was hardly available and certainly not forthcoming (208). Hygienic conditions were poor and death rates high. Under these conditions, in 1923 the population had shrunk by 45%; in some parts of Greece no children were born to refugee parents during an entire year. Such social and physical hardships might well have contributed to the further spread of hashish use among this large minority population. During the years that followed, hashish use persisted despite proscriptive legislation. The retail price was low, making it accessible to many (196).

From 1932 to 1970 the narcotics laws of Greece became increasingly severe. Until the end of the civil war in 1950, the laws were not strictly enforced and hashish use flourished. After this date, there was a gradual decrease in the illegal cultivation and use of hashish. The latest version of the law, which is enforced, can be summarized as follows: A drug addict must be confirmed as such by designated officials of the government medical service. Such an addict is then considered sick and subject to "attenuating circumstances" in the court trial required by law. As an addict, he is given a lighter sentence than the nonaddict. Punitive and corrective measures that may be imposed by the courts include imprisonment from 1 to 10 years, fines ranging from 50,000 to 10,000,000 drachmas ($1,500 to $300,000), deprivation of a driver's license for at least 2 years and up to life, confiscation of private property where the drug was found, dishonorable discharge from the armed forces, and prohibition of foreign travel.

Yet the men identified in this study continue to use hashish, despite its proscription. They apparently become known to the police, the courts, and medical authorities, and a symbiotic relationship seems to have evolved. To the extent that they continued to cooperate in these and other experimental studies for which permission was granted by government officials, they are assured of protection by the medical authorities involved in the study during the investigation period.

Sample Selection and Methods

2

Selection and Definition of Users and Controls

Aris Liakos, Demitra Madianou, Costas Ballas, and
Costas Stefanis

The selection of subjects for the user sample and appropriate controls was a critical phase in these studies. Cannabis use is illegal in Greece and uncommon among youth. Chronic users represent a subculture of older men, segregated from the rest of the population by their commonality of origins, residence, and social relationships. Unbiased sampling and properly selected control groups are essential to evaluate the effects of chronic cannabis use on mental and physical health and social functioning of the users. That many factors may influence the results is evident from the comparison of the observations in recent controlled studies (11,20,73) which fail to confirm earlier reports in which these requirements were not met (13,17,30,107).

SELECTION OF USERS

For many years long-term hashish users had been under study at the University of Athens, and members of this population were referred to us by Professor C. Miras, Chairman of the Department of Biochemistry. The subjects were familiar with research procedures and were willing to participate in the study. From these users, additional subjects were identified and included in the study.

During the summer of 1971 the research team examined cannabis users and established relationships with them. The social worker and psychiatrists visited the neighborhoods where the subjects lived, met their families, and were able to resolve most suspicions derived from their longstanding difficulties with the authorities. Other cannabis users became known during these visits and were persuaded to come to the hospital for examination. Through these contacts and those with local authorities (Town Hall, social agencies, police, etc.) the reported data were checked and verified. Users were paid a fee of approximately $15 for their participation in this phase of the study.

Cannabis users thus were derived from two main sources: They were referred by Professor Miras or were recruited from the community. Subjects were included in the study group if they met the following selection criteria:

1. Cannabis had been used for more than 10 years at the time of examination.

2. No other addictive substances were used, with the exception of alcohol. Alcohol use was a reason for exclusion only in cases where subjects got drunk regularly, could not do without alcohol, and their drinking habits interfered with their work performance.

3. There was an absence of incapacitating physical illness.

4. The maximum age was 58 years.

By summer 1972, 60 cannabis users were examined; of these, 39 had been referred and 21 recruited. Of the 39 referred, 11 were excluded: 4 subjects were older than 58; 3 had used heroin; 3 were classed as alcoholic; and 1 subject reported the use of amphetamines. Of the 21 users recruited by us, 19 were included in the study group. Two subjects were excluded: one was not using hashish regularly (present use) and the other reported the use of LSD. The final sample of 47 cannabis users included 28 referred and 19 recruited.

The users referred by Dr. Miras differed from the recruited group in some measures. Their mean age was higher (44.3 compared with 35.4 years; $t = 3.29, p < 0.01$); the mean years of use was higher (26 compared with 18.8 years; $t = 2.64, p < 0.01$); and they reported longer abstinence periods (9.44 compared with 3.35 months; $t = 2.01, p < 0.05$). More subjects from the referred group were residents of Tavros, a defined area where immigrants are concentrated (64.28% compared to 10.52%; $\chi^2 = 13.38$, $p < 0.001$); and a smaller proportion came from other parts of Athens (14.28% compared to 47.36%; $\chi^2 = 6.19, p < 0.02$). In medical examinations the incidence of palpable liver was higher in the referred group (seven subjects compared with one; $\chi^2 = 3.92, p < 0.05$). In other tests the two groups were not different, and for our purposes the subjects are treated as one sample.

Subjects came to the laboratory at Eginition Hospital (the neurological and psychiatric facility of the University of Athens) to be assessed for their suitability for inclusion in the study. Each subject was examined on a separate day beginning at 9 a.m. and continuing until approximately 2 p.m.; the following sequence of procedures was employed:

Time	Procedure
0:00	Psychometric testing: progressive matrices
0:30	Social history
1:30	Physical examination
1:40	Psychometric testing: WAIS
2:35	Psychiatric interview
3:30	Lunch
4:00	Neurological examination
4:15	Electroencephalogram
5:15	End of procedure

SELECTION OF CONTROLS

The methods and procedures employed for selecting controls were the same as for cannabis users. After each user was examined, he was asked to send a male friend or neighbor of similar age who would like to come to the hospital and have a "check up" similar to the one he had. Some controls were also recruited from the community in the same way as cannabis users were. Users and controls received the same fee ($15) for participating in the examination.

The criteria described above for the selection of users were also employed for controls, except for criterion 1, which refers to cannabis use. In the case of controls only subjects who never smoked cannabis (even once) were included, and subjects who reported use of other addictive substances with the exception of alcohol were excluded.

During 1971–1972, 64 subjects who seemed suitable for inclusion in the group of controls were examined; 24 were recommended by the hashish users and 40 were recruited. Forty controls were included in the final sample (9 referred by users and 31 recruited). Twenty-four were excluded for the following reasons: eight had smoked hashish on several occasions; five were alcoholic; four were older than 58 years of age; three were not tobacco users; two had a recognizable neurological disorder (myopathy and epilepsy); one reported the use of heroin; and one was a family member of a hashish user.

A comparison of the recruited controls and those referred by the users differed in that the men referred by the users were less educated (3.44 years of schooling versus 5.90 years; $t = 2.61$, $p < 0.02$) and the mean number of job changes were higher (4.0 versus 2.76; $t = 2.04$, $p < 0.05$). In other measures the two groups were similar, and they were combined for further study.

MATCHING

The sample of cannabis users was not random in the statistical sense; a matching method was used to complete the sample of controls. The two samples were matched for age, sex, and the following factors believed to influence the measures under study:

Tobacco use: All cannabis users were tobacco smokers. Tobacco is traditionally mixed with hashish by Greek users. This is done because hashish is very concentrated and too solid to be smoked in pure form. Since tobacco smoking may cause respiratory ailments, controlling for this variable was considered necessary, and smoking at least 10 cigarettes per day was a criterion for inclusion in the control group.

Alcohol use: Heavy users of alcohol were excluded. Using a four-point scale of alcohol use (0 = no use; 1 = use to 4 glasses wine a week; 2 = to 1 bottle wine a week; 3 = to 1 bottle wine a day; and 4 = greater than one bottle a day), the hashish users scored 0.80 ± 1.07 and the controls scored 0.77 ± 1.02 units. No alcohol use was reported by 58% of the controls and by 48% of the hashish users.

Socioeconomic status: The sample of cannabis users belonged to a low socioeconomic group, as evidenced by their residence, profession, and income. Most cannabis users lived in areas previously assigned to Greek refugees from Asia Minor, and a large proportion had refugee parents. This factor could be associated with the habit of cannabis use, and matching for it was considered desirable. Low social class is related to increased rates of mental disorder and thus provided a further basis for matching on this factor. By selecting controls from the same residential areas, subjects of approximately the same socioeconomic status could be selected. However, residence alone does not guarantee proper matching. Most cannabis users were born and raised in this environment, and this may have played a precipitating role in their hashish initiation. Therefore controls were matched for both *residence at birth* and *place of upbringing*. Residence of the family at the time of the subject's birth was defined as residence at birth. Place of upbringing was considered the residence of the subject from birth to 15 years of age. In cases where the subject did not reside at the same place during this time, the place where the subject spent the major portion of this period was considered the place of upbringing.

Education: The two groups were also matched on education, which may otherwise have influenced psychological test performance.

Because the number of parameters for matching was large and the time and number of controls limited, a subject-to-subject matching was not possible. Therefore the groups were matched for age, and statistical differences between the two groups were tested for the remaining parameters (Table 2-1). No differences were found except for the number of tobacco cigarettes smoked per day. Cannabis users reported smoking an average (mean ± SD) of 38.22 ± 17.5 cigarettes per day in comparison with 26.75 ± 14.43 cigarettes per day for the controls ($t = 3.34$; $p < 0.01$). However, since there was no difference between the two samples in the incidence of respiratory system disorders (Chapter 5), failure to match the samples on this factor was not considered significant.

The final sample consisted of 47 chronic users and 40 nonusing controls matched for age, socioeconomic status, education, and residence.

REPRESENTATIVENESS OF USER SAMPLE

To determine the representativeness of the hashish user (experimental) sample, an epidemiological and sociocultural profile of the reported hashish-using population in Greece was obtained. This information is based on data generated from the official Greek narcotic archives. The general hashish-using population is compared to the total Greek population and to the experimental sample.

TABLE 2-1. *Composition of controls and hashish users*

Criteria	Cannabis users (N = 47)		Controls (N = 40)		t	p
	Mean ± SD		Mean ± SD		t	p
Age	40.72 ± 12.12		41.72 ± 7.6		0.52	ns
Education	4.22 ± 2.86		5.37 ± 2.69		1.93	ns
Tobacco (cigarettes per day)	38.22 ± 17.5		26.75 ± 14.43		3.34	<0.01
Refugee parents	No.	%	No.	%	χ^2	p
Father	20	42.55	24	60.0	0.31	ns
Mother	23	48.93	24	65.0	1.06	ns
Both	17	36.17	21	52.5	2.34	ns
Residence at birth						
Area A (Tavros)	6	12.76	10	25.0	2.15	ns
Area B (Petralona)	10	21.27	9	22.5	0.01	ns
Area C (Peristeri)	13	27.45	6	15.0	2.02	ns
Area D (other parts of Athens)	14	19.78	13	32.5	0.07	ns
Area O (Asia Minor)	4	8.51	2	5.0	0.41	ns
Upbringing						
Area A	16	34.04	20	50.0	2.26	ns
Area B	11	23.4	7	17.5	0.45	ns
Area C	12	25.52	5	12.5	2.33	ns
Area D	8	17.02	8	20.0	0.12	ns

Data Sources

A search of the archives of the narcotic units of the Athens metropolitan police, the Piraeus metropolitan police, and the Athens suburban constabulary was undertaken. These archives encompass information for all of Greece with the exception of the city of Patras and the island of Corfu. The records studied cover the period 1958–1973.

Methodology and Methodological Problems

The archival search was conducted by a psychiatrist and a social worker who systematically collected data in the headquarters of the three narcotic units. Each unit devised its own system of record-keeping, so that any given drug abuser may have a record in two or even all three units. Adding to the complexity, the archives of each unit include different kinds of information, and the range of the information recorded by each unit may vary depending on the time period during which they were collected. Most records, however, contain the following data: name and surname, nickname, parents' name, place of birth, date of birth, place of residence, occupation, and illegal activities other than those on file.

Only the oldest files of one unit provide data such as starting age and events associated with initiation to hashish smoking. Some files include information about imprisonments, although most include only dates of arrest for drug abuse without mentioning if the user was released after identification or remanded for trial. In some instances the records cite "drug abuser" without indicating the type of drug used. In such cases the researchers who had established good working relations with the narcotic squads, discussed the question in detail with the police officials. In the few cases where only ambiguous or incomplete information was available, the records were excluded from the study.

After this process, all usable records (5,589) were compared and cross-referenced so that one final card, as complete and inclusive as possible, was generated for each drug abuser. Of the 5,589 records, 1,893 were duplicates, leaving 3,696 as the data pool. Subjects were classified by drug used and were identified as hashish users only if they were utilizing this substance exclusively. Of the 3,696 drug users, there were 3,021 males and 107 females who used only hashish; 330 were heroin addicts; 52 used other drugs such as amphetamines or barbiturates; and 186 were foreigners arrested in Greece.

Since the experimental sample of the study included only males, women were excluded from the archival analysis. Individuals arrested in Greece but residing permanently abroad were also excluded. Of 3,021 males classified as exclusive hashish users, 125 had incomplete records. As no standard classification of socioeconomic status in Greece existed, categorization of the subjects' status was determined according to educational background, occupation, and place of residence. On this basis, five categories were generated: high status, middle status, working class, engaged in illicit activities and dependent, peasantry. With regard to places of birth and residence, subjects were allocated into nine geographic areas. The Department of Attika was separated from the rest of central Greece as it includes the two major urban centers, Athens and Piraeus.

RESULTS

The study attempted to analyze, despite the limitations, the data from the police archives concerning the total hashish population of Greece; to compare the characteristics of the hashish population to the general population based on the 1971 census; and to compare the experimental sample of hashish users to the total hashish user population.

During the past 20 years Greece has become an industrial nation; the proportion of the agricultural population has shifted from 55% to 35%. This has been accompanied by the large-scale movement of people from rural to urban areas, primarily to Greater Athens including Piraeus, which now contains one-fourth of the entire population of Greece. The urbanization process appears to be even more significant for hashish users, as revealed by a comparison of places of birth and current residence of the total hashish population. In the region of Athens, for example, the locally born hashish-using population is 50% less than the provincially born hashish-using population which migrated to the urban center. A striking finding is that the incidence of hashish users in the borough of Tavros (Greater Athens) has increased during the last decade from 0.39% to 2.54% (Table 2-2).

By contrast, the hashish-using population of the provinces has been greatly reduced. In the Peloponnesus, the proportion of users has dropped from 17.6% to 4.8%, and in Epirus from 3.8% to 0.3% (Table 2-2). (It is unclear if the movement of rural-born hashish users into Athens means the gravitation of already socialized users to a center of hashish traffic or if the urbanization process was instrumental in initiating the practice of hashish use.)

Users of hashish tend to concentrate in and about Athens: the borough of Tavros has the highest concentration of hashish users (0.5%), compared to Piraeus with an incidence of 0.1% and Athens proper with 0.1% (Table 2-3). Thessaloniki in Macedonia and Kalamata in the Peloponnesus have a relatively high incidence of hashish users, 0.02% and 0.01%, respectively. These latter figures can be attributed to the fact that the two provincial centers are port cities.

Analyzing the total hashish population by socioeconomic status (Table 2-4) reveals that hashish users are predominantly in the working class (61.6%). A high proportion are unemployed or are supported by underground activities (21.4%). A similar proportion (12.7%) belong to the middle class, while the peasantry (4.1%) and higher class (0.1%) supply the smallest number of hashish users.

TABLE 2-2. *Distribution of the hashish users population according to place of birth and residence*

| | | Hashish population | | | |
| | General population (No.) | Place of birth | | Place of residence | |
Area		No.	%	No.	%
Department of Attica	2,797,849	1,175	38.89	2,323	76.89
Region of Athens	2,101,103	628	20.78	1,378	45.61
Borough of Tavros	15,795	12	0.39	77	2.54
Region of Piraeus	439,138	395	13.07	633	20.95
Rest of Dpt. of Attica	257,608	152	5.03	235	7.77
Rest of Central Greece	734,469	156	5.16	53	1.75
Peliponese	986,912	531	17.57	146	4.83
Ionian Islands	184,443	74	2.44	11	0.36
Epirus	310,334	38	3.77	9	0.29
Thessaly	659,913	114	1.25	57	1.88
Macedonia	710,352	192	6.35	128	4.23
Thessaloniki	345,799	88	2.91	76	2.51
Thrace	329,582	40	1.32	18	0.59
Aegean Islands	417,813	188	6.22	41	1.35
Crete	456,642	124	4.10	46	1.52
Asia Minor		216	7.14	—	—
Abroad		32	1.05	26	0.86
Unknown		100	3.31	163	5.93

TABLE 2-3. *Incidence of hashish users in the general population*

Area	General population	Hashish No.	Hashish %
Department of Attica	2,797,849	2,323	0.082
Region of Athens	2,101,103	1,378	0.065
Borough of Tavros	15,795	77	0.48
Region of Piraeus	439,138	633	0.14
Rest of Dept. of Attica	257,608	235	0.09
Rest of Central Greece	734,469	53	0.007
Peloponese	986,912	146	0.014
Ionian Islands	184,443	11	0.005
Epirus	310,334	9	0.002
Thessaly	659,913	57	0.008
Macedonia	710,352	128	0.008
Thessaloniki	345,799	76	0.021
Thrace	329,582	18	0.005
Aegean Islands	417,813	41	0.009
Crete	456,642	46	0.010
Abroad at present	—	26	—
Unknown	—	163	—
Total population of Greece (1971 census)	8,768,641	3,021	0.032

TABLE 2-4. *Socioeconomic status of hashish population*

Socioeconomic status	Total hashish population (N = 2,628) No.	Total hashish population (N = 2,628) %	Males (N = 2,488) No.	Males (N = 2,488) %	Females (N = 107) No.	Females (N = 107) %
High	3	0.11	3	0.11	—	—
Middle	335	12.74	326	12.94	9	8.18
Working	1,619	61.60	1,599	63.50	20	18.18
Unemployed, dependent, underground, etc.	562	21.38	452	17.95	77	70.00
Peasantry	109	4.14	108	4.28	1	0.90

TABLE 2-5. *Job level of males by origins*

Job level	Refugees (%)	Migrants (%)	Athenians (%)
Unskilled	7	5	1
Semiskilled	27	40	33
Skilled	27	23	29
Petty proprietor	29	6	7
Lower white collar	4	10	12
Independent artisan	5	9	9
Middle white collar	1	7	9
Total No.	84	123	111

TABLE 2-6. *Occupation and marital status of the two populations*

Parameter	General population of Greece		Total hashish population of Greece		p
	No.	%	No.	%	
Occupational status					
Employed	4,268,639	95.1	2,066	78.62	0.001
Unemployed	219,941	4.9	562	21.38	0.001
Total	4,488,580		2,628		
Marital status					
Married	2,182,140	48.61	370	50.00	ns
Divorced, separated, cohabiting	44,660	0.99	72	9.86	0.001
Widowed	483,200	10.75	0	—	0.001
Single	1,776,580	39.58	298	40.14	ns
Not declared	2,000	0.06	—	—	—
Total	4,488,580		740		

Eva Sandis, an American sociologist who studied Nea Ionia, a refugee community in Attika (167), found that occupational levels of refugees from Asia Minor, migrants of rural Greece, and Athenian respondents are lower for refugees than for migrants and Athenians (Table 2-5). Her findings are in accord with the present data, since it was found that the rate of unemployment among the hashish users (21.4%) was higher than that of the general population (4.9%) ($p < 0.001$).

Comparing the total hashish-using population to the general population with regard to marital status (Table 2-6) revealed significant differences in

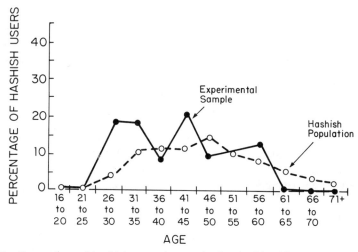

FIG. 2-1. Percentage of hashish users by age in the total hashish-using population in Greece and in the experimental hashish sample.

the percentages of "divorced, separated, and cohabiting" and the "widowed" categories ($p < 0.001$), and no differences in the "married" and "single" categories. The two populations also show differences in education. Hashish users are less educated (5.06 years of schooling, ± 3.64) than the general population (5.49 ± 3.45 years; $p \leq 0.01$).

A comparison of ages in the total hashish-using population and the present experimental sample finds no difference between distribution of the two (Fig. 2-1). The total hashish population had a mean age of 44.5 years, and the sample 40.7 years. The total hashish population was more educated than the experimental sample. The mean years of schooling are 5.06 ± 3.64 for the total hashish population and 4.22 ± 2.86 for the experimental sample ($p \leq 0.01$). This difference is best explained by the fact that the experimental sample consisted primarily of lower-working-class people.

Specifics on hashish smoking were available in the police archives for only a limited number of users (142 cases). Comparison of these data with those of the experimental sample focused on the starting age of hashish smoking and the years of use. The mean starting age for the total hashish population is 23.5 ± 7.05 years whereas for the experimental sample it is 17.61 ± 4.12 ($p \leq 0.001$). No difference exists for years of hashish use between the two populations, with 24.2 years as the mean for the total sample and 24.3 years for the experimental group.

We may conclude that hashish users in Greece are derived primarily from the working class and are differentiated from the general population with regard to age and education. On the other hand, our experimental sample is representative of the lowest urban working class and is differentiated from the total hashish population of Greece by lower levels of education and earlier starting ages for the smoking of hashish. Differences between our experimental sample and the total hashish population may be attributed to the selection criteria imposed by clinical objectives, which restricted admission to the research project to heavy chronic users only while the total hashish-using population of Greece exhibits various degrees of use—from very occasional to heavy.

SUMMARY

The procedures employed for the selection of the users and controls of the study are outlined. Satisfactory matching was obtained for sex, age, refugee origin, residence at birth, alcohol use, and upbringing (place of residence to the fifteenth year of age).

3

Methods of Acute Inhalation Experiments

Rhea Dornbush, John Boulougouris, Jan Volavka, and
Anna Kokkevi

Experimental studies of marijuana have focused on the effects of acute use. A typical paradigm involves the administration of single doses of marijuana (usually up to 20 mg THC-Δ-9 when smoked) with observation of behavior thereafter (usually up to 1 hr, although longer periods have been studied). The effects of marijuana are compared to the effects of placebo, administered usually several days apart.

Because the emphasis is on acute inhalation, these effects are well defined. The physiological and behavioral effects are rapid in onset, changing during the course of measurement and returning to baseline rapidly (51). There is an increase in heart rate (46,47,90,159), an increase in the abundance of EEG alpha activity, and a decrease in average EEG frequency. Both EEG and heart rate effects peak early in the postsmoking period and then decrease (193).

The effects on performance in perceptual, cognitive, and motor tasks vary. A decrement is sometimes obtained (33,188) or there is no change (51,189). Short-term memory is most consistently impaired (1,49). Subjective effects are described as "pleasant" and tend to persist after objective changes are no longer measurable (134).

The effects of smoking marijuana and other cannabis substances were observed in Greek hashish users to determine if the long years of use altered their immediate response compared to the immediate responses of occasional, short-term users. The design and many procedures in this study were similar to those used in experiments performed on young adult American users (21–30 years of age).

METHODS

Subjects

Twenty users were studied. Their age (mean ± SD) was 43.0 ± 10.4 years, and the duration of use was 18.8 ± 8.7 years. This is a subsample of the original study group and did not differ from that group in their age, years of use, duration of abstinence periods, and mental test performance.

Drugs

As there is some evidence that all cannabis preparations do not have similar effects even though they may have equivalent THC-Δ-9 concentrations, three preparations were used: marijuana, hashish, and purified THC-Δ-9. The marijuana, THC-Δ-9, and placebo were supplied by the U.S. National Institute on Drug Abuse (NIDA) and contained 2.6% THC-Δ-9. Hashish was of Greek origin with an average 4.5% THC-Δ-9 content.

Subjects smoked different preparations of cannabis, with amounts of THC-Δ-9 ranging from 0 to 180 mg (Table 3-1). These preparations were mixed with tobacco and rolled into large cigarettes with an appearance identical to those the subjects usually smoked.

Procedures

The testing took place within 5 days; 4 days were consecutive, and the fifth occurred after an interruption of at least 1 day. This sequence was prompted by the delayed arrival of purified THC-Δ-9 at the Athens laboratories. The order of drug administration was only semirandom: marijuana, two doses of hashish, and placebo were completely randomized, but THC-Δ-9 was always the last condition. The order of administration was considered in the statistical analyses.

Subjects were examined individually; two were seen each day—one in the morning and one in the afternoon—and they underwent the procedures described in Table 3-2. The specific technique for each measure is described in each section presenting the results. Continuously recorded variables (e.g., EEG, heart rate, temperature, and respiration) were recorded on an eight-channel polygraph. Some measures were also recorded on a Hewlett-Packard 4-channel FM tape recorder for computer analyses in New York.

Data Processing

Multiple stepwise linear regression analyses were performed (35). The order in which variables are entered into these regression equations was determined by the investigators. This makes the regression analyses almost

TABLE 3-1. *Content of smoked cannabis samples*

Sample	Source	THC-Δ-9 content (mg)
Placebo	U.S. marijuana leaf, THC-Δ-9-free	0
Marijuana	U.S. leaf	78
Hashish (low conc.)	Greek hashish, 2 g	90
THC-Δ-9	Liquid infused on placebo (U.S.)	100
Hashish (high conc.)	Greek hashish, 4 g	180

TABLE 3-2. *Acute procedures*

Time	Duration (min)	Procedure
0:00–0:20	20	Galvanic skin response (GSR) and pupil measurement
0:20–0:50	30	Electrode placement and connection; checking instruments
0:50–1:05	15	Evoked potentials
1:05–1:15	10	Presmoking period recordings, including EEG, pulse rate, respiration, temperature, and finger plethysmography
1:15–1:30	15	Smoking period recordings, including EEG, pulse rate, and temperature
1:30–2:00	30	Postsmoking recordings, including EEG, pulse rate, respiration, temperature, finger plethysmography, and "high" self-ratings by the subject
2:00–2:25	25	Interval during which the following measurements were recorded: pupil size, psychological test battery (digit span, *barrage de signe,* star tracing, time estimation, serial sevens), evoked potentials
2:25–2:45	20	Postinterval recordings including EEG, pulse rate, respiration, temperature, finger plethysmography, and "high" self-ratings
2:45–2:55	10	Psychological test battery
2:55–3:15	20	GSR and pupil measurement
3:15–3:25	10	Questionnaire administration
End of procedure		

identical to analyses of covariance. In all analyses, effects of the intersubject variance were accounted for prior to investigating other relationships.

To determine the effect of the nonrandom assignment of THC-Δ-9 as the last condition, analyses of some variables (EEG parameters and heart rate) were performed twice. In one analysis the observations with all five substances were included and order effects were not accounted for. In a second analysis the THC-Δ-9 sessions were excluded and order effects were accounted for. In this second set the effects observed during session 1 differed significantly from those during session 4 in several instances but did not affect the relationship between the variables being studied. The differences between sessions 1 and 4 suggest a "first-session effect" or habituation to the experimental situation. As the relationship among variables was not affected, the remaining analyses included THC-Δ-9 and excluded order of sessions. However, as is discussed in Chapter 11, the order of sessions, particularly the occurrence of THC-Δ-9 as the last condition, may indeed have affected performance in the psychological test battery.

4

Methods of Withdrawal Study

Rhea Dornbush, Aris Liakos,
and Anna Kokkevi

The systematic studies of the development of tolerance or the effects of a forced marijuana abstinence in long-term users are few. Two strategies have generally been employed to demonstrate the effects of repeated use of marijuana. One involves the administration of marijuana to subjects classified on the basis of frequency and duration of use (11,66,126,145,200). Differences in behavior as a function of differences in use are determined. Mendelson et al. (126) studied casual and heavy users of cannabis during 21 days of daily marijuana consumption. Casual users were defined as those with a 2- to 5-year history of use, smoking marijuana 1–12 times a month. Heavy users also reported 2–5 years of use, but they had been smoking daily for at least 1 year prior to the study. This classification was similar to that used by Perez-Reyes (175), who defined frequent users as those smoking marijuana several times a day for at least 1 year prior to the study, and infrequent users as those using less than one cigarette per month.

In the second strategy, marijuana is administered daily for brief periods to subjects with a common frequency in duration of use. To date, the period of daily administration has varied from 10 to 52 days (111,159,205). Placebo periods precede and follow smoking days. In these studies the target period is typically the period of marijuana use, with emphasis on changes in behavior during the smoking period rather than changes from use to nonuse or nonuse to use (50).

Recent studies suggest that there may be a differential development of tolerance to the behavioral, physiological, and subjective effects of marijuana, and that this may be related to the frequency and duration of use (91,200). Mendelson et al. (126) found that both casual and heavy users increased their marijuana consumption during 21 days of daily smoking, but only the heavy users exhibited tolerance for the physiological and subjective effects. The reduction in effect was evidenced more in its duration rather than its intensity. It is even more difficult to demonstrate the development of tolerance on psychological test performances. With repeated administration of standard doses, psychological test performance improves with time (50), but it also improves with increasing consumption over time (111, 126).

In many North American experimental studies of marijuana, the subjects do not fit the criterion of long-term use, which has been defined as 10 years or longer (111,134). The subjects are usually regular or infrequent users for, more typically, 1–5 years. As most subjects are 18–30 years of age, with most starting their use of marijuana during late high school or college, the population of long-term users is small and poorly identified. In instances where long-term users are identified, they are frequently multidrug users. To determine long-term effects uncontaminated by the use of other substances, investigators have sought populations beyond North America, i.e., in Jamaica, Costa Rica, and Greece, where cannabis use has been culturally accepted for decades, if even only among small groups within the population at large. In the present study of long-term Greek hashish users, an examination of abstinence symptoms after the cessation of marijuana use was undertaken. Although the experimental periods of smoking and withdrawal were each of the 3 days' duration, we were able to observe under laboratory conditions the effects of the abrupt cessation of use and the consequences that abstinence has on physiological, behavioral, and mood responses when marijuana is again consumed.

METHODS

Subjects

Sixteen users served as subjects. All were part of the original study group of 47 users (Chapter 2), and 9 had also participated in the experimental study of acute use. The mean age ($\pm$ SD) of the 16 subjects was 40.8 ± 9.00 years, and the mean years of hashish use was 24.6 ± 9.00 years. The characteristics of this subsample did not differ from the characteristics of the original study group.

Smoking

Each subject smoked twice a day. All smoking periods were 30 min in duration. Smoking was *ad libitum*. An adequate supply of ready-made cigarettes of marijuana or placebo were placed in front of the subject; he was instructed to smoke as much as he pleased. Each cigarette contained tobacco and either 1g of active marijuana or placebo material.

Drugs

The active material was marijuana supplied by the U.S. National Institute on Drug Abuse (NIDA) and contained 2.6% THC-Δ-9. Thus each marijuana cigarette contained 26 mg THC-Δ-9. The placebo, also supplied by NIDA, was free of cannabinol and other cannabinoids.

Procedures

Subjects were hospitalized for six consecutive days. Prior to hospitalization, subjects came to the hospital twice a day to smoke marijuana *ad libitum* (Saturday and Sunday). They were then admitted into a small, 15-bed ward for six consecutive days (Monday to Sunday morning).

Two subjects were investigated together during each week of the experiment. They followed a program of investigation that provided continuous staff observation during each 24-hr period. The daily program of investigation was arranged in such a way that although it was the same for all subjects it started 4 hr later for the second subject of the pair; i.e., the program for the first subject started at 8:45 a.m. and for the second subject at 12:45 p.m.

The 6 days of investigation were divided into two periods: a period of marijuana smoking (3 days) and a period of placebo smoking (3 days). Eight subjects followed the placebo-marijuana order (order 1) and eight the marijuana-placebo order (order 2), as indicated in Table 4-1. The crossover design was employed to control for learning and hospitalization effects.

Test Periods

There were several evaluation periods after the first and second smoking. Measurements employed to assess withdrawal effects were performed 2–4.5 hr after the first smoking. These measurements were recorded on all experimental days, i.e., days 1–6 unless otherwise indicated. Measurements to assess acute effects of smoking were performed after the second smoking and usually on only 1 day of each 3-day period. The tests and time of administration are shown in Table 4-2.

First Smoking

On each day, immediately after smoking, estimates of the "high" achieved were reported on a 10-point scale. The Greek word for this high is *mastura*. At the same time, subjects were required to indicate the price they were willing to pay for what they had smoked (in drachmas, the monetary unit in Greece; each drachma is approximately 3¢).

TABLE 4-1. *Smoking format of withdrawal study*

Format	Days 1–3	Days 4–6
Order 1 (subjects 1–8)		
First smoking	Placebo	Marijuana
Second smoking	Placebo	Marijuana
Order 2 (subjects 9–16)		
First smoking	Marijuana	Placebo
Second smoking	Marijuana	Placebo

TABLE 4-2. *Testing schedule for the 6-day withdrawal study*

Time (min)	Procedure	Day[a]					
		1	2	3	4	5	6
0–30	*First smoking*	X	X	X	X	X	X
35	Mastura ("high"), price willing to pay	X	X	X	X	X	X
120	Clinical ratings	X	X	X	X	X	X
	Blood pressure	X	X	X	X	X	X
130–160	Psychological test battery	X	X	X	X	X	X
210	Neurological examination	X	X	X	X	X	X
225	Structured psychiatric interview	X		X	X		X
240	EEG	X	X	X	X	X	X
	Heart rate	X	X	X	X	X	X
	Mastura ("high")	X	X	X	X	X	X
	Respiration	X	X	X	X	X	X
	Temperature	X	X	X	X	X	X
	Plethysmography	X	X	X	X	X	X
	Evoked potentials		X			X	
270	Pupil size			X			X
270–300	*Second smoking*	X	X	X	X	X	X
300–305	Pupil size		X			X	
305	*Mastura* ("high"), price willing to pay	X	X	X	X	X	X
	Psychological test battery			X			X
	Heart rate		X			X	
	Mood		X			X	
	Respiration		X			X	
	Temperature		X			X	
	Plethysmography		X			X	
335	Evoked potentials		X			X	
360	Biochemical samples			X			X

[a]For subjects in order 1: days 1–3 were placebo days and days 4–6 were marijuana days. For subjects in order 2: days 1–3 were marijuana days, and days 4–6 were placebo days.

Clinical ratings

Two hours after each smoking, self-ratings were recorded on a point scale for *mastura*, anxiety, depression, restlessness, fatigue, and irritability. Additionally, subjects were clinically assessed for constipation, flatulence, abdominal pain, cramps, and appetite. Flatulence, abdominal pain, and cramps were assessed as present or not, while appetite and constipation were assessed on a three-point scale: more than usual, as usual, less than usual. After these assessments the blood pressure was measured in standing and lying positions.

Psychological testing

At 2 hr 10 min after the first smoking, the psychological test battery was administered; this testing required 30 min. The tasks are described in Chapter 11. They included serial sevens, *barrage de signe* (an attentional task), time estimation (of a 5-min task), digit symbol substitution test (DSST), and number ordination.

Neurological examination

The neurological examination was performed 3.5 hr after smoking. The following items were examined: reflexes (corneal, tendon), vibration sense, finger-nose test, big toe test, walking on line test, dysdiadochokinesia test, Romberg test, turn, nystagmus, and speech test.

Structured psychiatric interview

The psychiatric interview was conducted 3 hr 45 min after smoking on the first and third day of each 3-day period (i.e., days 1, 3, 4, and 6). It contained the following items taken from form A of the Mental Status Schedule Examination (173): (a) body image (questions 57–61, 63), and one question was added: "feel strong and able to help all others"; (b) imagination (questions 85–87); (c) perceptual distortions (questions 88–90); (d) bodily sensations (question 92); (e) auditory hallucinations (questions 117–119); (f) quality of speech (question 186); quantity of speech (questions 207–210); and (h) rate of speech (questions 211 and 212). A five-point rating scale for suspiciousness was also added to the structured psychiatric interview.

Physiological and subjective measurements

Physiological and subjective measurements were recorded approximately 4 hr after the first smoking. These measurements involved a 30-min continuous, or nearly continuous, recording of EEG, heart rate, respiration rate, temperature, and plethysmograph. *Mastura* was also rated every 10th minute during the 30 min of observation. Evoked potentials were included in the physiological testing on the second day of each sequence (i.e., days 2 and 5). Pupil size measurements were included in the physiological testing on the third day of each 3-day testing sequence (i.e., days 3 and 6).

Second Smoking Period

On each day, immediately after smoking, *mastura* and price willing to pay were recorded.

Physiological and subjective measurements

On the second day of each 3-day smoking period (i.e., days 2 and 5) physiological and subjective measurements were recorded during the 30 min immediately following smoking. The EEG was not measured.

Psychological testing

On the third day of each 3-day smoking period (i.e., days 3 and 6) the psychological test battery was administered immediately after smoking.

Data Processing

On each day of marijuana smoking, the subjects smoked a different number of cigarettes. They usually smoked less each succeeding day, less after the second smoking period than after the first, and less in order 2 (marijuana-placebo) than in order 1 (placebo-marijuana). These data are described in Chapter 16. To account for the effects of smoking different quantities of THC-Δ-9 in the different experimental conditions, covariance analyses are appropriate; the covariate is the number of cigarettes. However, two factors mitigated against our use of covariance. The analysis of variance of the covariate (cigarettes) resulted in a significant "sequence by drug" interaction. Significant interactions in the covariate violate the assumptions underlying the use of covariance analysis. Secondly, a more important factor is whether the different amounts of THC-Δ-9 consumed in the various experimental conditions would result in different responses. For instance, if greater amounts of THC-Δ-9 did not result in greater increments in heart rate than lesser amounts of THC-Δ-9, this would suggest the development of tolerance. For these reasons analyses of variance were performed to permit assessment of effects as they varied with THC-Δ-9 quantity.

Depending on the specific data, either three-way or two-way analyses of variance were performed. After the first smoking, the following data were incorporated into separate three-way analyses of variance: each task of the psychological test battery, EEG (separate analyses were done for each frequency band), heart rate, respiration, temperature, plethysmograph readings, blood pressure, *mastura*. The physiological recordings were usually continuous for 30 min, and an average was obtained for each variable. Order (placebo-marijuana, marijuana-placebo); drug (placebo, marijuana), and days (1, 2, 3) were the main variables. In these analyses the order by drug interaction permits a determination of whether the drug was administered first (days 1–3) or second (days 4–6).

For the physiological data, after the second smoking three-way analyses were performed. Order, drug, and time (5, 10, 15, 20, 25, and 30 min) were the main variables. For these data the recording period was immediately after smoking and was usually continuous for 30 min. Five-minute averages were obtained. Time is included in these analyses as there may be greater fluctuations immediately after smoking than 4 hr after smoking, when the principal effects have decreased. The data incorporated in this design were heart rate, respiration, temperature, and plethysmograph readings.

The psychological test data obtained immediately after the second smoking were evaluated in two-way analyses of variance. Order and drug were the main variables, and separate analyses were done for each task.

Mastura and drachmas were the only two variables that were recorded immediately after both smoking periods each day. Separate three-way analyses were performed on these two variables. Because placebo ratings for both *mastura* and drachmas were effectively zero, they were not included in the analyses. The three main variables in these analyses are order, day, and smoking period (first smoking, second smoking). The analyses and specific testing procedures for each measurement are reviewed in the chapters describing these measurements.

Results: Sample Characteristics

5

Characteristics of Hashish Users and Controls: Social, Family, and Personal

John Boulougouris, Aris Liakos, Demitra Madianou, and
Costas Stefanis

The development of an amotivational syndrome and family and personal psychopathology are said to distinguish marijuana users from nonusers (71–73). Psychosocial differences between marijuana users and nonusers have been demonstrated in college students based on questionnaire evaluations (79). Brill and Christie (20) reported that marijuana users experience more difficulty in deciding on career goals and that they leave college slightly more frequently (than nonusers) to reassess their goals. However, no association between marijuana use and psychosocial disorder was demonstrated. Chopra (30) suggests that the distinction must be made between occasional, regular, and moderate users, and those who indulge in excess. The latter category of users are more prone to exhibiting adverse psychoclinical effects.

Users in the United States and Canada belong mostly to the categories of occasional and moderate users. In North America excessive cannabis use, like that of alcohol, has been attributed to preexisting personality problems (98). In Jamaica and in the sample of users in Greece, where marijuana use is part of the cultural experience of the user, this may not be the case. In a study of Jamaican users, Rubin and Comitas (166) failed to discriminate users from controls on measures of social functioning, identifiable psychopathology, criminality, social and economic mobility, and the use of other drugs. In these users cannabis-seeking behavior is considered a function of a long complex of social experiences.

As part of the study of the sample of hashish users in Greece, social and family characteristics were compared with those of the nonuser group. The characteristics included drug history, family and social factors, work performance, and patterns of everyday life experience.

REVIEW OF METHODS

The criteria for the selection of hashish users and controls is presented in Chapter 2. The data presented in this chapter were obtained in a semistructured psychiatric interview following the format of Mayer-Gross et al. (120).

33

The social history was obtained by a social worker. The reported hashish data (i.e., starting age of hashish smoking, years of smoking, frequency and quantity of smoking during the past and present, as well as the periods of abstinence) were obtained by the psychiatrist and the social worker. "Past use" was defined as the period before 1967, a year during which law enforcement increased and hashish consumption decreased. The period from 1967 up to the day of the interview (1971) was defined as "present use."

The psychiatric interview focused on the family's mental health, family relationships, presence of a broken home (i.e., loss of parent by death or separation before the subject reached the age of 15), and abnormal psychopathology preexistent to hashish smoking. A special effort was made to define any relationship between criminal behavior and hashish smoking.

The social worker recorded the occupational status, the reasons for job changes, and, apart from the data on hashish smoking, the use of other related substances including alcohol. The psychiatrist's and the social worker's interview each lasted approximately 1 hr. In addition, the social worker visited the homes of some hashish users ($N = 29$) and some controls ($N = 13$) to interview the wives and occasionally other members of the families. The final comparison is made between 47 hashish users and 40 controls.

RESULTS

Reported Hashish Data

The mean age of onset of cannabis smoking was 17.61 ± 4.12 years, and the subjects had smoked nearly every day for 23.1 ± 9.7 years (Table 5-1). The mean frequency of smoking each day was 4.5 ± 3.76 times in the past and 2.32 ± 1.01 times in the present. Users consumed a mean quantity of 7.48 ± 5.98 g hashish per day in the past and 3.13 ± 1.81 g/day recently. The mean number of abstinence periods for various reasons (imprisonment, difficult to obtain, etc.) was 1.21 ± 1.01, and the mean duration of such periods was 10.06 ± 10.84 months. Chemical analysis of hashish samples described by the subjects as of "average strength" revealed a 4–5% content of THC-Δ-9. On this basis, users were currently smoking the equivalent of an average of 140 mg THC-Δ-9 per day.

The main reasons for initiating hashish use were curiosity (22 subjects of the 47 examined), conformity and pressure (19/47), and for therapeutic reasons (6/47). Five subjects claimed that they started smoking hashish to stop their use of alcohol and that the substitution was successful. No significant life events were associated with hashish initiation.

Subjects claimed to continue smoking for relaxation (13 subjects), euphoria (12), better work (9), habit (6), and to increase sexual desire (2),

TABLE 5-1. *Reported hashish data*

Parameter	Starting age	Years of use	Times/day on day of smoking		Quantity on day of smoking (g)		Abstinence periods	
			Past use	Current use	Past use	Current use	Times	Total duration (mo)
Mean	17.61	23.10	4.5	2.32	7.48	3.13	1.21	10.06
SD	4.12	9.70	3.76	1.01	5.98	1.81	1.01	10.84

while some could verbalize no reason (9). The main reasons for decreasing their recent drug use were fear of the law (17 subjects), financial reasons (9), and lack of available hashish (8). Six subjects smoked daily before going to work, 2 after work, and 16 before and after work; 13 did not relate their smoking to work. Thirty subjects preferred to smoke with company; 10 preferred to smoke alone; 6 indicated that either with company or alone was satisfactory; and 1 did not state a preference.

Personal and Family Characteristics

No significant differences were found between hashish users and controls in age, education, and number of occupations and job changes (Table 5-2). Both populations were poorly educated, although controls had one more year of schooling than the users. Of 47 hashish users, 6 were illiterate, 34 attended school for 1–6 years, and 7 had a secondary education. Of 40 controls, 3 were illiterate, 28 attended school for 1–6 years, and 9 had a secondary education.

Hashish users and controls belonged to the lower socioeconomic group. Occupationally the hashish users were mainly peddlers, flower or fruit street sellers, scrap metal collectors, and flayers in slaughterhouses. The controls were mainly skilled factory workers or small-business owners. The main reasons for job changes reported by hashish users were better salary and difficulties in getting along with their employer. The controls changed jobs to obtain better working conditions and for permanent positions.

TABLE 5-2. *Personal history data*

Parameter	Cannabis users (N = 47) (Mean ± SD)	Controls (N = 40) (Mean ± SD)	t	p
Age	40.72 ± 12.12	41.72 ± 7.6	0.52	ns
Education	4.22 ± 2.86	5.37 ± 2.69	1.93	ns
No. of occupations	3.10 ± 1.67	3.07 ± 1.78	0.08	ns
No. of job changes	3.74 ± 2.14	4.55 ± 2.44	1.63	ns

The two populations did not differ in the presence of neurotic traits during childhood or in being separated from either parent before age 15. No differences were found in marital status.

The wives of 24 hashish users approved of their husbands' smoking hashish. They claimed hashish smoking was calming and improved sexual interest and performance. Fifteen wives disapproved of hashish smoking because of the social stigma and expense.

Examining the family history of mental illness, more hashish users (five) had mentally ill mothers than did the controls (one), but this difference was not statistically significant. Although more hashish users had alcohol- or cannabis-using fathers, these differences were also not significant (Table 5-3).

Significant differences were found in the following personal history data (Table 5-4):

Previous psychiatric treatment: Nine hashish users (19%) had previous psychiatric treatment compared with two (5%) of the controls ($\chi^2 = 3.94, p \leq 0.05$).

Regular military service: Only 26 of the 47 cannabis users (55%) had served in the regular army, compared with 38 of the 40 controls (95%). This difference was significant ($\chi^2 = 17.4, p < 0.001$). The main reasons for exemption from military service were reported cannabis use and antisocial behavior.

Imprisonment: Twenty-five cannabis users (53%) had been in prison because of cannabis law violations in comparison with one (3%) of the controls ($\chi^2 = 26.5, p < 0.001$). The one control subject was sentenced for hashish possession and not for hashish use. Additionally, 29 cannabis users (62%) were sentenced for reasons other than cannabis violations in comparison with 10 (26%) of the controls ($\chi^2 = 11.76, p < 0.001$).

TABLE 5-3. *Family history data*

Family history	Cannabis users (N = 47)		Controls (N = 40)		χ^2	p
	No.	%	No.	%		
Refugee parents						
Father	20	42.55	24	60.0	0.31	ns
Mother	23	48.93	24	65.0	1.06	ns
Both	17	36.17	21	52.5	2.34	ns
Family history of mental illness						
Father	0	—	1	2.5	—	ns
Mother	5	10.63	1	2.5	2.22	ns
Siblings	7	14.89	3	7.5	1.16	ns
Alcoholic father	14	29.78	9	22.5	0.59	ns
Cannabis-user father	3	6.38	1	2.5	—	ns
Broken home	14	29.78	5	12.5	3.78	ns

TABLE 5-4. *Personal history data (significant differences)*

Personal history	Cannabis users (N = 47)		Controls (N = 40)		χ^2	p
	No.	%	No.	%		
Previous psychiatric treatment	9	19.14	2	5.0	3.94	0.05
Regular military service	26	55.31	38	95.0	17.49	0.001
Imprisonment						
Related to cannabis	25	53.19	1	2.5	26.49	0.001
Other reasons	29	61.70	10	26.0	11.76	0.001
Skilled workers	12	25.53	25	62.5	12.08	0.001
Unemployed when examined	20	42.55	6	15.0	7.82	0.01

Work record: Although the two samples did not differ in number of occupations and job changes, more cannabis users were unemployed when seen (43%) than controls (15%). This difference was significant ($\chi^2 = 7.82$, $p < 0.01$). Similarly, 12 cannabis users were skilled workers (26%) compared with 25 (63%) of the controls ($\chi^2 = 12.08$, $p < 0.001$).

The amount of reported hashish smoking was not correlated either with type of employment (skilled or unskilled), prison sentences due to reasons other than cannabis law violations, or employment when these subjects were seen. Mental illness was not clearly related to the amount of hashish smoking.

DISCUSSION

The data concerning hashish use were retrospectively reported by the subjects, and their validity and reliability may thus be questioned. The subjects, however, are confirmed long-term users and have not contaminated their smoking with other psychoactive substances. The hashish data were obtained from two independent interviewers—the psychiatrist and the social worker—and were confirmed in interviews with wives or other close relatives. The amount of THC-Δ-9 consumed is difficult to estimate because of the variability of potency as well as weight and size of hashish cigarettes. The concentration of THC-Δ-9 in hashish samples obtained from the men was 4–5%. In the United States typical users consume marijuana with a 0.5–1.5% THC-Δ-9 content. The reported amount of hashish use by Greek users is similar to other reports from Eastern countries (171).

The reasons for initiating hashish smoking may differ from those described in Western societies (45), but curiosity and conformation are common, powerful motives. The threat of law was the main reason for reduction, which is in agreement with other findings (200), and not changes of marriage and entry into parenthood as have been suggested (76).

Examination of the control population showed that the two populations were well matched on the selected criteria. It is therefore unlikely that the initiation of hashish smoking is due to nonspecific environmental or cultural factors since the control subjects were brought up in the same communities as the hashish users (Chapter 2) and did not differ in their family characteristics. That naive users may imitate their parents who smoke was not supported by the present findings. The family characteristics of hashish users agree with the findings in chronic ganja users in Jamaica (11); i.e., the degree of family psychopathology is not related to hashish smoking.

The differences in amount of sustained employment and its type among the subjects may appear as evidence of an "amotivational syndrome" in the cannabis smoker (122). However, since hashish smoking is disapproved, considered deviant, and involves severe prison sentences, the differences in employment may be related to these factors. On the other hand, hashish users had more imprisonments (than the controls) due to reasons other than hashish. The greater incidence of prison sentences in hashish users is not related to the higher incidence of antisocial behavior or to the severity of hashish smoking. This difference may be attributed to the fact that these individuals were known to the police because of their hashish use and were more susceptible to arrest. Most of these arrests were for theft.

SUMMARY

The two populations were similar on the demographic variables for which they were matched. They differed in military service and number of imprisonments, differences that may have been the result of hashish use. They also differed in previous psychiatric treatment, degree of skill in work, and employment at the time of the interview.

6

Subjective Experiences of Cannabis Use in Long-Term Users

Aris Liakos and John Boulougouris

A variety of subjective effects of cannabis have been reported. Most descriptions include pleasant mood changes (12,164), but unpleasant effects are also reported (16,68,98,99,197). Factors that influence the subjective effects of drugs include the user's personality and expectations, the dose of cannabis, the setting, and prior experience. These individual factors and the often anecdotal and uncontrolled study methods may account for the variations in the reported subjective effects (98).

The methods of observation affect the nature of the reports. In some studies the subjects report their experience immediately after the use of cannabis (21,83,121,129,164,198); in others they report retrospectively while not under the influence of the drug (69,75,183). Both methods utilize unstructured interviews (69,75) or structured self-report measures (83, 183,198).

Roth (165) points out that techniques to assess subjective effects which are administered during intoxication concentrate on the drug-produced changes that are only a fraction of the total psychic effects of the drug, whereas questionnaires administered when the subject is not under the influence of the drug may provide greater insight into why people use drugs.

In the present study subjective effects were reported by chronic users at various times during the study period: immediately after smoking as nonstructured interview responses; structured, questionnaire-type self-reports; self-ratings; and retrospectively, at times when chronic users were free from the short-term effects of cannabis. The subjective effects reported in this chapter are retrospective.

METHOD

During the course of the psychiatric evaluation, subjects were asked three main questions: In what way does cannabis smoking affect you? What do you feel after smoking? Does it have any unpleasant effects? The examiner elaborated on these three questions for clarification, if required. The subjects' reports were recorded verbatim and were later analyzed under several headings, which are shown in the tables containing the results. Results are divided in two main categories: usual and generally pleasant effects, and undesirable effects. The effects were reported by 45 of the sample of 47 chronic cannabis users described in Chapter 2.

RESULTS

The results are shown in Tables 6-1 and 6-2, divided into those considered pleasant and those considered unpleasant. Table 6-1 shows the usual and generally experienced pleasant effects, which were reported by most subjects. The commonest effects are dry mouth, increased sexual arousal, euphoria, overtalkativeness, laughter, increased appetite, and relaxation.

These effects were reported by more than 50% of the subjects. The majority of the effects are related to elevated mood (euphoria, talkativeness, laughter, relaxation, ideas of superiority). Other effects concern memory (both increased and decreased recall), perception (enhanced perception, floating sensation), thinking (ideas of superiority, thoughtfulness, slow thinking), and performance (working better, driving better). There are also some somatic effects (dry mouth, increased appetite, and increased sexual desire). No subject reported all the effects in any session. Two subjects (4%) reported as many as 10 effects occurring; 22 (50%) reported seven to nine of the effects; 20 (44%) reported four to six; and only one (2%) subject reported as few as three.

Unpleasant effects are cited in Table 6-2. Undesirable effects are reported by fewer users and are experienced less frequently than the desirable effects. Smokers related these adverse effects to excessive doses or to very potent materials. The commonest symptoms were panic attacks, persecu-

TABLE 6-1. *Usual and "pleasant" effects of cannabis smoking (N = 45)*

Effect	No. of subjects	%
Dry mouth	43	95.6
Increased sexual appetite	40	88.9
Euphoria	⌐35	77.8
Talkativeness	31	68.9
Laughter	30	66.7
Increased appetite	28	62.2
Relaxation	23	51.1
Improved work	20	44.4
Feeling of superiority	17	37.8
Improved problem-solving	12	26.3
Enhanced perception	10	22.2
Floating sensation	8	17.8
Increased recollection	7	15.6
Decreased recollection	4	8.9
Improved driving	2	4.4

tory ideas, and thought block, each reported by 20% of the su~~~~
sion, psychomotor retardation, dizziness, illusions, and hallucinations were
each reported by 8–15% of the subjects. The remaining symptoms concern
somatic effects (palpitation, sweating, disorders of sleep, vomiting, agitation) and inability to work, and each were reported by under 5% of the
subjects. Of the 16 effects considered undesirable, four to six were reported
by 3 subjects (7%), whereas no unpleasant effects were reported by 19
(41%). One effect was reported by 10 subjects (22%); two effects were
reported by 8 (17%); and three effects were reported by 7 (15%).

There was an increase in the number of reported pleasant or desirable
effects with increases in the number of undesirable effects; i.e., those
subjects who reported no unpleasant effects reported a mean of 5.8 pleasant
effects, whereas those subjects who reported the occurrence of three unpleasant effects reported a mean of 8.0 pleasant effects.

DISCUSSION

Most subjects reported pleasurable effects after smoking. Emotions,
thought, memory, perception, and motivation were each affected by cannabis. There is a relative lack of reports of subtle perceptual effects (e.g.,
changes in time perception or "insight" experiences), but this may reflect
the lack of sophistication and the use of special terminology by the chronic
users. These men are poorly educated and have special expressions to
describe their experiences that are difficult to understand or to translate.

It is sometimes difficult to understand why subjects continue to smoke
when they report undesirable effects from it. However, for these long-term

Greece
education, socioeconomic status, and occupational ... associate ganja with clear-thinking, meditation and concentration, euphoria, feelings of well-being, good feelings toward others, and self-assertiveness (166). While users maintain that ganja enhances their ability to work, their daily work is tedious manual labor, which marijuana somehow makes more tolerable, as may be the case with the Greek users.

7

Psychological Test Characteristics of Long-Term Hashish Users

Anna Kokkevi and Rhea Dornbush

Information on the effects of long-term cannabis use is very limited. Until recently studies of long-term and/or moderate use were typically based on surveys or clinical observations. The study samples included multidrug users, prisoners, and/or psychiatric patients. For example, Williams et al. (205) conducted studies with pyrahexyl (judged qualitatively similar to marijuana) and marijuana. The subjects were prisoners; the potency of marijuana was not assayed; and there was no control group. Psychological measurements indicated that comprehension and analytical thinking were made more difficult, and an adverse effect was noted in accuracy on those tests which required concentration and manual dexterity. Soueif (170) studied Egyptian users; his sample included more than 800 prisoners, 60% of whom were illiterate. Users were slower learners than controls and did significantly worse on objective tests of mental performance. However, a significant number of users also used other substances, especially opium. There was a positive correlation between the duration of hashish use and the use of opium, and drug users tended to seek agents acting on the central nervous system (CNS) more than nonusers did.

Campbell et al. (26,27), using pneumoencephalograms, demonstrated the existence of cerebral atrophy in cannabis users (Chapter 9). Subjects were multiple-drug users or were known to have a history of brain damage. Kolansky and Moore (106) suggested the presence of a specific pathological response in the CNS to cannabis, basing their view on uncontrolled clinical experience. Marijuana use was high in their sample of 13 subjects identified over a 6-year period, suggesting the existence of a preexisting severe personality disorder. Subjects who indulge in excess may be unstable and susceptible, and are more prone to adverse psychoclinical effects (31). Miras (130) reported that very heavy hashish users demonstrated EEG abnormalities and mental deterioration, although these findings have not been confirmed (57,58).

Recent studies of mental functioning are more systematic and methodologically precise. These studies, with two exceptions (studies in Costa Rica and Jamaica), are on the effects in as-yet short-term users. Grant et al. (66) studied medical students who were moderate, regular users of marijuana for at least 3 years. Compared with a control group of nonusers, there were no differences in functioning in a large battery of neuropsychological tests. Hochman and Brill (79) surveyed college users. Chronic use was defined as three times per week for 3 years or daily use for 2 years. Chronic use of marijuana in this group was not accompanied by deterioration in functioning or adaptation.

In a study of Jamaican users who were daily consumers of marijuana for at least 10 years, there were no differences in psychological test performance between users and an adequately matched group of controls (18). The test battery included assessments of perceptual-motor functioning, memory, and concept formation.

In a sample of users in Costa Rica (who smoked daily for an average of 17 years), there were no differences between users and nonusers on neuro-psychological, intelligence, or personality tests, nor were there relationships between the level of daily use and test performance (168).

Discounting the studies with significant methodological deficiencies (which appear mainly related to the type of subject selected), the effects of marijuana on mental performance detected in chronic users are related to acute use and are transient. Disturbances in mental functioning during acute cannabis intoxication have been amply documented (49).

SELECTION OF PSYCHOLOGICAL TEST INSTRUMENTS

The Wechsler Adult Intelligence Scale (WAIS) and Raven Progressive Matrices 30 (PM) were used to assess general intelligence and mental functioning in Greek users (156,157,199). In addition, subtests of the WAIS were used to evaluate the possibility of impairment in specific cognitive and perceptual functions. The WAIS has not been standardized on a Greek population, but long experience (by the research team) with a translated and adapted form used in the psychiatric hospital at Athens University Medical School encouraged its use in this study. The Raven Progressive Matrices, considered a more "culture-free" test of intelligence than the WAIS, was administered at the same time to provide additional information about the reliability and validity of the WAIS results.

These tests were administered to 47 users and a control group of 40 nonusers matched for age, sex, demographic region, socioeconomic status, education, and consumption rates of alcohol. None of the users were tested while under the acute influence of hashish, although some had smoked several hours before the examination (most had smoked the day before).

BEHAVIOR DURING TESTING

The hashish users were sensitive to the fact that their mental capacities were being evaluated. They tended to be defensive and to excuse their test performance because of inadequate education. No other behavioral differences were observed during the testing period between the user and nonuser groups. Most of the subjects were interested, attentive, and cooperative during the testing sessions and maintained a high level of motivation.

RESULTS

Statistical data for the two samples of subjects are presented in Table 7-1. The intelligence quotients (IQs) derived from the two tests (WAIS and PM) are similar in both groups. The correlations between the total WAIS and PM scores for the hashish group is 0.60. The correlation of performance IQ (PIQ) with PM is 0.66 and that of verbal IQ (VIQ) with PM is 0.58. For the control group the correlations were: total WAIS and PM, 0.70; PIQ and PM, 0.71; VIQ and PM, 0.60. All correlations were significantly different than zero ($p < 0.001$). These correlations of a nonverbal "culture-free" test (the PM) with the WAIS (a verbal test not standardized in Greece) permits a fair degree of confidence in the use of the adapted WAIS in this sample.

The IQ scores on the WAIS and PM classify both controls and users in the "dull-normal" range. The low educational level (mean years of schooling for users was 4.22, and for controls 5.37) and low socioeconomic status contribute to this finding (199).

There were no differences between users and controls in their total IQ or PIQ scores. Controls performed significantly better than users in three subtests: Comprehension, Similarities, and Digit Symbol Substitution. The control group obtained a higher VIQ than the users ($p < 0.05$). This finding is due

TABLE 7-1. *WAIS and progressive matrices (PM) results*

Test	Cannabis users (N = 47)		Controls (N = 40)		t	p
	(Mean ± SD)		(Mean ± SD)			
PM IQ	83.81	9.31	86.57	11.16	1.22	ns
IQ total	83.70	11.91	88.38	11.67	1.83	ns
IQ verbal	87.41	10.80	92.62	12.48	2.04	0.05
IQ performance	80.98	13.13	85.59	12.46	1.66	ns
Information	7.49	2.58	8.46	2.51	1.76	ns
Comprehension	8.53	2.67	10.05	2.38	2.79	0.01
Arithmetic	9.19	1.91	9.33	1.96	0.33	ns
Similarities	6.34	2.84	8.15	2.59	3.09	0.005
Digit span	7.17	2.14	6.87	1.95	−0.68	ns
Vocabulary	8.93	1.69	9.46	2.04	1.29	ns
Digit symbol	6.49	2.01	7.39	2.11	2.01	0.05
Picture completion	7.68	2.50	7.82	2.64	0.25	ns
Block design	7.40	2.43	8.10	2.68	1.25	ns
Picture arrangement	6.57	3.05	7.77	3.10	1.79	ns
Object assembly	6.38	2.72	7.38	2.46	1.79	ns

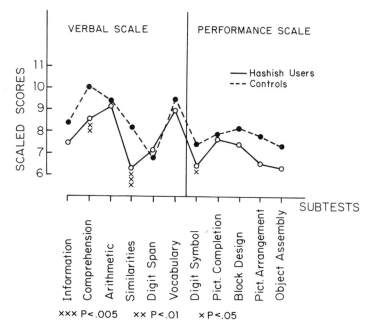

FIG. 7-1. Scaled scores for each subtest on the WAIS for the hashish users and controls.

to the higher scores of the controls on two subtests of the verbal scale (Similarities and Comprehension) (Fig. 7-1).

In American populations differences between VIQ and PIQ greater than 12 points are considered evidence of deterioration or diffuse brain damage (209). In the Greek sample, for both users and controls, the differences between the PIQ and the VIQ was 7 points. Experience with the WAIS in Greece on normal populations reveals systematic differences between PIQ and VIQ of approximately 7 points (VIQ > PIQ). These observations do not provide evidence of deterioration of mental abilities in the hashish users.

DISCUSSION

The differences between controls and users on the three subtests of the WAIS (Comprehension, Similarities, DSST) may be related to the incidence of mental illness in the user group (Chapter 8). It is known that sociopaths and psychotics have impaired judgment and impaired abstract thinking abilities (Comprehension and Similarities). However, a comparison of two subgroups of the users—the mentally ill and the normal) did not demonstrate a difference in performance in these subtests. Comprehension assesses the degree of social acculturation, particularly in the sphere of moral or ethical judgment (209). Hashish use in Greece is deviant, and differences in comprehension between users and controls may represent the users' poorer acculturated status.

The Similarities subtest is a test of abstraction or concept formation. Difficulties in abstraction are often related to faults of adaptation rather than to limitations of reasoning ability. This may be the case with the user group, particularly if one accepts the interpretation of the deficit in Comprehension; i.e., deficits in the two subtests may be related more to acculturational and adaptational processes than to logical reasoning abilities. These differences may also be related to the lower education level of the hashish users (4.22 years) than the controls (5.37 years), although the difference in education is not statistically significant: Poorer performance by the users on the Digit Symbol Substitution Test may also reflect their recent use of hashish, as the test was given within two hours of smoking hashish by some users. This interpretation is made more plausible by the greater pulse rates in the users. These were measured just before the psychological tests were administered (Chapter 10). Beyond this, it is difficult to interpret the differences in subtest performance between user and control groups.

Neither the WAIS nor the Progressive Matrice scores are evidence of mental deterioration or organicity in the chronic hashish users. Subjects in both user and control groups have a dull-normal intelligence level, a finding that correlates with their low educational level and socioeconomic status. The verbal-performance score differences are small, and the same degree of difference is present in both groups.

The sample studied in Jamaica had similar socioeconomic status but a slightly higher mean educational level, although the percentage of illiteracy was higher (Jamaica 43%, Greece 12%). It is possible that the detection of subtle intellectual dysfunctions in groups with initially low levels of mental functioning are less easily observed. Satz (168) suggests that a "floor effect" may occur in populations such as those studied in Jamaica and Greece. If the tests are too difficult, then depressed performance levels may mask differences between groups. Satz, however, did not find evidence for a floor effect in a sample of Costa Rican users, although their mean educational level was higher than in either the Jamaicans or the Greeks (eighth grade).

8

Incidence of Mental Illness in Hashish Users and Controls

Costas Stefanis, John Boulougouris, and Aris Liakos

The relationship between chronic cannabis use and psychiatric illness is complex. It is widely believed that an acute transitory psychotic state may occur immediately after use under certain conditions. However, no causal relationship between use and prolonged illness has been demonstrated (62). Where psychiatric illness has been associated with heavy cannabis use, it is unclear whether the psychopathology is antecedent to, consequent to, or coincidental with use (70,101,128,135).

A number of studies originating mainly from Eastern countries describe an association of chronic cannabis use and mental disorder (5,13,17). Other studies relate cannabis use to the inception of a specific mental syndrome (30,178). For example, Kolansky and Moore (106,107) reported a specific pathological organic CNS response to marijuana. Severe symptomatology followed the onset of marijuana use in adolescents and young adults, and disappeared after discontinuation of drug use. However, sampling bias, methodological inadequacies, and anecdotal data in these studies limit their usefulness.

Representative samples of chronic cannabis users who do not use other addictive substances are difficult to obtain, and factors likely to influence the incidence of mental disorder are hard to control. Moreover, there has been considerable difficulty in establishing an accurate diagnosis of mental disorder on the basis of the currently employed clinical criteria. The following classification was recently recommended (135):

Acute panic anxiety reaction: Symptoms are usually exaggerations of normal cannabis effects and subside with reassurance or when the drug effects have worn off.

Acute brain syndrome (toxic delirium): This syndrome most frequently occurs at high doses and includes clouding of mental processes, disorientation, confusion, and marked memory impairment; it subsides when the drug effects have worn off.

Prolonged reactions: These include psychotic reactions, flashbacks, and the amotivational syndrome.

Nonpsychotic, prolonged adverse reactions: These include changes in life style.

Employing more vigorous methodological criteria than previously reported, Halikas et al. (70) surveyed 100 regular marijuana users and 50 controls. The duration of marijuana use was slightly more than 2 years. There was a high lifetime incidence of psychopathology in both user and nonuser control groups, although sociopathy was found in a greater number of users than controls. However, diagnosed psychiatric illness preceded the use of marijuana. Halikas suggests that the use of marijuana may reflect a higher incidence of acting-out behavior.

Hochman and Brill (79) surveyed users and nonusers on the college campus and found no difference in the incidence of mental disorders between groups. These studies employed users whose duration of use is relatively short. Beaubrun and Knight (11), on the other hand, compared cannabis users who had had daily consumption for at least 7 years with nonusing controls. There were no differences between the two groups in incidence of mental illness, alcoholism, abnormal mood, abnormal thought processes, or abnormal behavior. Similar studies of chronic users in Costa Rica failed to document differences between users and nonusers (34).

Among the populations studied, the Greek sample has the longest documented duration of daily use (approximately 25 years) uncontaminated by other psychoactive substances. Their mental status was compared with appropriately matched nonusing controls ($N = 47$ and 40, respectively).

The assessment of mental health of the subjects and their final diagnosis was made by the consensus of three psychiatrists participating in the study. It was based on information obtained from a structured social history taken by a social worker, a psychiatric examination performed in a semistructured way following the Mayer-Gross et al. (120) format, and the data gathered from home visits, reports of local civil authorities, and records of subjects who received psychiatric treatment prior to the study. The diagnostic criteria of the American Psychiatric Association (44) were used for the diagnostic evaluation of this information.

RESULTS

Significantly more users (38%) than controls (18%) were diagnosed as suffering from a psychiatric abnormality (Table 8-1). Twelve users were diagnosed as having "personality disorders" (26%), compared with three of the controls (8%). There is also a significant difference in the incidence of the subcategory of personality disorders of the antisocial type. Five users were diagnosed as having a personality disorder, antisocial type (11%), compared with none of the controls.

The incidence of other types of psychiatric abnormalities does not differ in the two groups. Three cannabis users (6%) and three controls (8%) were classed as neurotic, and one control was suffering from depression. Three users were diagnosed as psychotic, paranoid-schizophrenic type—they expressed loosely organized paranoid delusions unrelated to their drug intake.

TABLE 8-1. *Incidence of psychiatric disorders*

Type of disorder	Hashish users (N = 47)		Controls (N = 40)		χ^2	p
	No.	%	No.	%		
Personality disorders	12	25.53	3	7.5	4.94	<0.05
Antisocial type	5	10.63	0	—	4.51	<0.05
Other types	7	14.98	3	7.5	1.16	ns
Neurosis	3	6.38	3	7.5	0.04	ns
Depressive illness	0	—	1	2.5	—	ns
Schizophrenic disorder (paranoid)	3	6.38	0	—	—	ns
Total	18	38.28	7	17.50	4.56	<0.05

They neglected themselves and showed lack of insight. One of the three reported visual and auditory hallucinations; two had a positive family history of mental disorder. All three began their use of cannabis during their teens, with the onset of the psychotic symptoms many years later. One subject did report symptoms that may have had a psychotic basis at the age of 14. The diagnosis of an organic psychosis was not entertained for any user in this sample.

To investigate the relationship between the incidence of psychiatric disorders and the amount of cannabis consumed daily, the sample of users was categorized into two groups according to their mean use of hashish. Heavy users were defined as those who reported cannabis use above the mean daily consumption of the group, and moderate users as those who reported present use as lower than the mean daily consumption. There was a tendency for a negative relationship between the degree of cannabis consumption and the incidence of psychiatric abnormalities; i.e., more psychiatrically abnormal users were found among moderate users (43%) than among the heavy users (21%). No relationship between degree of consumption and incidence of psychiatric abnormality, employment, and imprisonment records was found (Table 8-2). Regular military service was not included in the compari-

TABLE 8-2. *Various comparisons between heavy and moderate smokers (according to present use of hashish)*

Item	Heavy smokers (N = 14)		Moderate smokers (N = 32)		χ^2	p
	No.	%	No.	%		
Skilled workers	1	7.14	10	31.25	3.11	ns
Imprisonments due to other reasons	7	50.00	22	68.75	1.46	ns
Employed when seen	9	64.28	18	56.25	0.26	ns
Mentally ill	3	21.42	14	43.75	2.08	ns

son since psychiatric disorder is a reason for exemption from military service.

The psychiatrically ill and normal users were compared for those aspects which discriminated users from controls (Chapter 5). More psychiatrically abnormal cannabis users were sent to prison for reasons unrelated to cannabis offenses (83%) than were psychiatrically normal users (48%) ($\chi^2 = 5.8$, $p \leq 0.02$); the groups did not differ in other measures.

DISCUSSION

This study shows a higher incidence of psychopathology in the population of chronic hashish users in comparison with controls. The difference is due mainly to the prevalence of personality disorders, particularly the antisocial type of personality. Since similar psychopathology has been noted by others (73), the role of cannabis use in determining this difference must be considered. It is possible that individuals with an antisocial type of personality are more prone to cannabis use, especially in a particular social setting. Hashish smoking in Greece is illegal and carries severe punishment and social stigma. In this setting cannabis use may be considered a form of antisocial behavior more likely to occur in people with a personality disorder or those alienated from the cultural values of the community. Since most of the subjects started smoking at a very early age, assessment of presmoking personality is not possible. The possibility of chronic cannabis use exerting a modifying influence on the personality of the users cannot be excluded.

We could not document a relationship between psychiatric disorder and the degree of cannabis use. This is another reason to suspect that psychiatrically abnormal subjects are more likely to be found among cannabis users, rather than cannabis use being the cause for a psychiatric abnormality. The difference in imprisonment records between psychiatrically abnormal and normal users can be explained by the prevalence of personality disorders among users.

The occurrence of three cases of psychosis among cannabis users, although not statistically significant, raises the question of prolonged, chronic cannabis use leading to a psychotic state. The clinical features, however, of our three cases were indistinguishable from those of chronic schizophrenia, and the positive family history in two of them suggests that genetic factors may have played a prominent role. The absence of features of an organic dementia is consistent with the other measures of brain function in these subjects, suggesting that the prolonged use of cannabis is not associated with gross brain damage (174).

This sample of users belongs to the special cultural subgroup of the Greek population—the Greek refugees from Asia Minor, of low socioeconomic level, and living in certain underprivileged areas. The investigated sample is representative of Greek chronic users (Chapter 2). We conclude from this study that long-term cannabis use is associated with a high incidence of personality disorders, a finding that may be related to the prevailing legal and social variables of hashish use in Greece.

9

Medical Studies in Long-Term Hashish Users

I. Physical and Neurological Examinations

John Boulougouris, E. Antypas,
and C. P. Panayiotopoulos

Long-term cannabis use has been associated with hazards to physical health. Chronic bronchitis, asthma, and pulmonary fibrositis (75a), arteritis (175b), endocarditis (116a), and hepatotoxic effects (101a,116a) have been reported. Transient neurological manifestations such as fine tremor of the fingers (4,15), nystagmus (2,15,162), and sluggish pupillary reactions to light and accommodation (162) have also been cited after cannabis. Most studies, particularly those that report long-lasting effects, do not consider factors other than cannabis use which may be responsible for these effects. In this chapter, the results of physical and neurological examinations of long-term users and matched controls are reported.

METHOD

In selecting subjects for study, incapacitating physical or neurological illness and alcohol dependence were reasons for exclusion. Three users and two control subjects were excluded because their examinations were incomplete. The data of this study are from 44 users and 38 control subjects.

Physical Examination

Detailed history and physical examinations of respiratory, cardiovascular, and alimentary systems were carried out by the senior physician. Pulse rate, blood pressure, the presence of conjunctival injection, hoarseness of the voice, and uvular edema were recorded. The neurological examination was carried out by an experienced neurologist. Particular attention was paid to corneal reflexes, nystagmus, pupillary reactions to light and accommodation, tremor, tests of ataxia, tendon reflexes, and vibration sense.

Alcohol Use

A five-point rating scale was used to assess reported alcohol use. The scale points were defined: 0 = no use; 1 = infrequent use, up to 4 glasses of wine a week; 2 = moderate use, up to 1 bottle of wine a week; 3 = frequent use, up to one bottle of wine a day; and 4 = heavy use, more than one bottle of wine a day and occasionally drunk.

RESULTS

Thirteen cannabis users (29.5%) and six controls (15.8%) had signs of bronchitis (high pitched wheezing on auscultation) (Table 9I-1). The difference in

TABLE 9.1-1. *Medical findings in 44 long-term cannabis users and 38 matched controls*

	Users	%	Controls	%	X^2	P
1. Bronchitis	13	29.5	6	15.78	2.17	N.S.
2. Emphysema	2	4.5	1	2.63	—	—
3. Hoarseness of voice	4	9.09	2	5.26	—	—
4. Uvular oedema	5	11.36	1	2.63	—	—
5. Conjuctival injection	4	9.09	—		—	—
6. Enlarged liver	8	18.18	1	2.63	5.05	.025
	Mean	S.D.	Mean	S.D.	t	P
7. Number of cigarettes smoked (reported)	38.2	17.6	26.7	14.4	3.25	.005
8. Pulse rate	80.4	10.1	75.9	7.4	2.32	.025

incidence of bronchitis in the two samples is not statistically significant. In no case was bronchitis severe enough to interfere with daily work performance. There is also no difference in the incidence of emphysema, hoarseness of the voice, uvular edema, or conjunctival injection. Eight hashish users (18.2%) and two controls (5%) were found to have enlarged, palpable livers, a difference that is statistically significant (p ≤ .025).

To further examine the relationship between the incidence of enlarged liver and cannabis consumption, the users were divided into two groups: heavy users, those who reported smoking cannabis cigarettes above the mean amount, and moderate users, those who reported smoking below the mean amount. No relation between the degree of cannabis consumption and enlarged liver was found (Table 9I-2).

Alcohol consumption was also examined in relation to liver enlargement by dividing the users into moderate drinkers (scale scores 0 to 2) and heavy drinkers (scale score 3 and 4). The liver was palpable more often in heavy alcohol users (Table 9I-3).

TABLE 9.1-2. *Relationship of enlarged liver to degree of hashish use*

	Enlarged Liver		Normal Liver				
	N	%	N	%	Total	X^2	P
Moderate Users (Below the mean daily consumption)	5	16.66	22	83.34	27	0.14	N.S.
Heavy Users (above the mean daily consumption)	3	21.42	14	78.58	17		

TABLE 9.1-3. *Alcohol use and incidence of enlarged liver*

	Drinking < 2 Points (moderate)	Enlarged liver	%	Drinking > 2 Points (heavy)	Enlarged liver	%	X^2	P
Present use Hashish Users N = 44	39	5	12.82	5	3	60.	6.63	.01
Controls N = 38	37	2	5.40	1	0	—	—	—
Total	76	7	9.21	6	3	50.0	8.64	.005

Users smoked more tobacco cigarettes (38) each day than did the controls (26). This difference is statistically significant. Users also had higher pulse rates (80 beats per minute) in comparison with controls (75 beats per minute).

The neurological examinations did not differ in the two samples. One subject complained of occasional, transient vertigo when he lay down or got up suddenly. Two users were found to have reduced grip strength, one had brisk tendon reflexes and impaired vibration sense, one had a mild tremor of the tongue, and in another, the corneal reflex was absent. Nystagmus, tremor, abnormal pupillary reactions, and disorders of gait and coordination were not found.

DISCUSSION AND SUMMARY

The main findings are the tendency for the users to have more respiratory ailments and a significantly higher incidence of palpable livers. The difference in bronchitis is not significant and could be attributed to tobacco use, as the hashish users were heavier tobacco smokers than controls. The incidence of enlarged liver is associated with the degree of alcohol consumption and not with the degree of cannabis use. The present data agree with the findings of other controlled studies where liver function tests were performed and failed to demonstrate a connection between cannabis and liver damage (79a). We also failed to find any neurological abnormality related to cannabis use (4,15).

9

II. Clinical Electroencephalography and Echoencephalography in Long-Term Hashish Users

C. P. Panayiotopoulos, Jan Volavka, Max Fink, and Costas Stefanis

There are few reports on the effects of chronic cannabis use on the resting EEG, and the reports that are available are conflicting. Some investigators found EEG abnormalities they interpreted to be an indication of cerebral damage due to cannabis (27,130), and others reported no significant abnormalities in chronic hashish users (43,166).

Miras (130), examining the resting EEG records of chronic hashish users in Athens, found slow waves which could represent evidence of cerebral dysfunction. Campbell (27) compared the resting EEG of 11 patients with psychotic reactions attributed to cannabis use, 11 cannabis users without apparent psychiatric reactions, 29 patients with schizophrenia, and 10 patients with neurological diseases. He reported that the cannabis users exhibited a greater degree of EEG abnormality than the other groups. Ten of the 11 patients with psychotic reactions after cannabis showed an abnormal EEG, while 8 of 11 cannabis users without psychiatric disorders also showed an abnormal EEG. In the latter group, 4 subjects who took only cannabis had EEGs "compatible with epileptic disorders." However, it is difficult to accept these findings without some reservation. Two of the 11 patients with psychotic reactions attributed to cannabis use had a history of EEG abnormalities before taking cannabis. One had a history of migraine headache, and another had an epileptic EEG and was receiving antiepileptic medication. In addition, none of the subjects could be considered chronic hashish users as some had used it only once or twice, at some time before the EEG recording (2 months). The longest duration of cannabis use was 2 months. Six of the 11 subjects identified as cannabis users without psychotic reactions had used LSD and/or amphetamines as well as cannabis.

Other authors found no significant abnormalities in the EEG of chronic hashish users. Deliyannakis et al. (43) examined 25 chronic hashish smokers who smoked hashish for 1–9 years (average 53 months). They smoked one cigarette of hashish from 4 times a day to once every 2 weeks (an average of 22.5 cigarettes per month). The investigators found that 13 EEG records were normal, 10 were within normal limits (but with a relatively increased amount of theta waves in the temporal and posterior areas), and 4 were classified as mildly abnormal with high-amplitude, irregular theta waves.

In an extensive study of chronic ganja users in Jamaica (166), the EEG records of 30 chronic smokers were compared with 30 matched control subjects, and no differences were found. In the ganja group, 22 records were considered normal, 3 equivocally normal, and 5 showed some minimal to moderate abnormality. The results were similar in the control group: 19 records were considered normal, eight equivocally normal, and three had minimal to moderate abnormalities. It was noted that low-voltage records were more frequently seen in the ganja users than in the control population (16 and 10, respectively), but the difference was not statistically significant.

Using another method, Campbell et al. (26) reported "evidence of cerebral atrophy" shown by air encephalography in 10 patients with a history of consistent cannabis smoking (3–11 years). The subjects were male, with an average age of 22 years. Some had used LSD (one was admitted as an emergency for LSD overdose) and amphetamines. Two were possible epileptics, and one was receiving treatment for schizophrenia. Three of six patients who were studied with EEGs had abnormal records. Estimates of the size of cerebral ventricles by air encephalography found the lateral and third ventricles to be dilated, compared to 13 controls selected from a similar age group of patients with a normal air encephalogram and normal neurological examination. The transverse diameters of the anterior part of the third ventricle were 4.1 and 6.0 mm for control and patient groups ($p < 0.01$); and the posterior diameters were 4.7 and 6.7 mm. These findings are endorsed by Schwarz (169) who asserts that the mental changes consistent with cerebral atrophy can be demonstrated by the mental status examination and functional inquiry.

These findings were criticized on the basis of the selection of the controls (180), the suitability of patients, and the method (24). In Bull's view, "neuroradiologists have failed to assess the volume of cerebral ventricles accurately and to determine the upper volumetric limit of normal. . . . The argument presented by Campbell . . . would, I think, fail to convince neuroradiologists unless supported by morbid anatomical evidence" (24).

MATERIALS AND METHODS

EEGs were obtained in 46 of the 47 chronic cannabis users; one hashish smoker refused to have the examination. Forty matched healthy subjects were used as controls. (For the selection of controls, see Chapter 2.)

The International 10-20 system was used for placing the silver-silver chloride stick-on electrodes. The recording was made on an Elema-Schonander 16 channel EEG machine. The patients were supine with their eyes closed. The records were visually assessed by two experienced electroencephalographers, and some of the records were read by an additional two. The records were scored without knowledge of which came from the users and which from the nonuser controls. The records were classified according to the conventions used by clinical electroencephalographers into three groups: (a) within normal limits; (b) borderline (mainly records of low amplitude with a fair amount of diffuse theta activity and no paroxysmal or localized abnormalities); and (c) abnormal. (These records are described in the text.)

Echoencephalography, a method of estimating ventricular size by reflection of ultrasonic signals, was used to determine the diameter of the posterior portion of the third ventricle using a Siemens echoencephalograph system. Studies were done in 14 users and 21 controls who agreed to cooperate for this test.

RESULTS

EEG findings are shown in Table 9-1. There is no difference in the percentages of normal, borderline, and abnormal EEG records between the 46 chronic hashish users and 40 matched control subjects. In chronic hashish users, six EEG records were classified as borderline: two records were of very low amplitude with a moderate degree of diffuse theta activity; two were of high amplitude (the alpha rhythm was more than 50 μV) with a moderate amount of theta activity which in one subject was slightly more pronounced on the right side; and two records were of very low amplitude, with predominant fast activity and some theta activity.

Six borderline records were found in control subjects. Of these, four were of very low amplitude with a moderate amount of diffuse theta activity. Two were of moderate to high amplitude with a moderate amount of diffuse theta activity, and one showed some mild paroxysmal tendency during overbreathing.

Four clearly abnormal records were found in the chronic hashish users. Two records had a great amount of theta activity with a preponderance on the left; one showed diffuse theta activity; and one showed a burst of 5-c/s, high-amplitude theta waves in the left anterior temporal regions.

TABLE 9-1. *EEG findings*

EEG diagnosis	Controls (*N* = 40)		Chronic hashish users (*N* = 46)	
	No.	%	No.	%
Within normal limits	28	70.0	36	78.2
Borderline	6	15.0	6	13.0
Abnormal	6	15.0	4	8.8

Of the six abnormal records in the control subjects, all showed increased theta and a lesser amount of delta activity, which in one was more pronounced on the right, and in two pronounced on the left. In these records, some bursts of sharp or theta waves were also seen, mainly during over-breathing.

EEG records of chronic hashish users tended to have a higher amplitude than the records of control subjects. EEG signs of drowsiness were detected in 14 (35%) of the control records and in 13 (28%) of the user records.

Of the three chronic hashish users who showed psychotic reactions, one refused to have an EEG and the other two had records which were within normal limits. Of the four chronic hashish users who had abnormal records, only one had personality disturbances of a depressive character.

In Echo-EEG, not one of the 14 chronic hashish users exceeded a 7 mm width of the third ventricle. This is the upper limit of the width of the third ventricle in patients with otherwise normal air encephalograms, according to Lonnum (115). Furthermore, no statistical difference was found between the 14 chronic hashish users and 21 control subjects (6.6 ± 1.0 mm and 6.3 ± 0.7 mm, respectively).

CONCLUSION

We failed to find either an abnormality or a particular EEG change in the resting EEG records of chronic hashish users; similarly, the Echo-EEGs were within the normal range. We have no reason, on clinical or EEG or Echo-EEG data, to suggest that long-term hashish use produces an organic mental syndrome.

Results: Acute Experiments

10

Acute Subjective Experiences on Inhaling Different Cannabis Substances

John Boulougouris and Rhea Dornbush

The principal subjective effect of cannabis is to promote an altered state of consciousness which has come to be known as the "high" (12,165). There is no generally accepted definition of "high" and no rigorous way to measure it. The problem was summarized by the Canadian Commission of Inquiry into the Non-Medical Use of Drugs (111):

> It is often difficult to find descriptions of the subjective effects of marijuana that are free from value judgements. Many effects seem to take on good or bad connotations depending on the circumstances in which they occur, the personal attitudes of the individual undergoing the experience, and the orientation of the observer who is recording them. Moreover, since many of the significant psychological effects are intensely personal, the laboratory scientist often has little opportunity to make objective measurements, and must rely on subjective, introspective reports communicated verbally through a language system which is frequently inadequate.

While the Canadian Commission concludes that there is indeed a general "highness" factor that can be differentiated by regular users, they point out that the rationale for continued cannabis use among regular users is often more complex than the single desire to attain the "high:"

> Besides the production of the "high," the most frequently mentioned reasons for continued use are the attaining of pleasure or an improved mood; the relief of tension and depression or as an adjunct to relaxation; heightened awareness, perception, or sensitivity; increased sociability or fellowship; and to assist in introspective or reflective pursuits.

This wide range of effects represents the interaction of personality and set variables with the pharmacological effects of cannabis. The different subjective reports reflect the psychological experience of the users more than they reflect differences in cannabis substances or dose (68,81,200).

Several studies indicate that different degrees of "high" are attained in chronic and irregular users with similar doses (127,200). Many other studies fail to find a relation between past use and the reporting of the "high" (91,145).

Subjective effects have been measured in various ways; the differences in the reports are related to the methods used to define the experience. The most frequent type of assessment is based on questionnaires administered in a historical survey fashion to determine why subjects use cannabis (72,165,182). Questionnaires have also been administered to subjects during or immediately after intoxication (50). Several attempts have been made to quantify the subjective experience and determine its time course during intoxication. These measurements have been limited to the "high" (6) (Chapter 14) and require a self-rating based on a point scale. In one instance (193) subjects were requested to rate both the degree of "high" they had achieved and the pleasantness of the experience. "High" and pleasantness differed in their physiological correlates. The "high" showed a linear relationship to the amount of EEG alpha activity, average alpha frequency, and heart rate. Pleasantness was independent of EEG measures; it increased with heart rate up to approximately 100 beats/min and then decreased. The cannabis-induced states were less uniformly euphoriant than generally believed. However, the dose (20 mg THC-Δ-9) used in that experiment was larger than the ones used to achieve a "social high" (91,111). It is probable that subjects titrate themselves by ingesting quantities sufficient only to reach their desired mental or physiological state.

In other laboratory studies after the administration of either ingested or oral cannabis in doses of 2.5–210 mg THC-Δ-9 (92,102), reactions have varied from a sense of calm and well-being (50,68) to panic attacks, thought disorder, and other adverse reactions (124).

In the present study various methods were used to assess the subjective experiences of marijuana intoxication. The first was self-rating on a 10-point scale of *mastura* ("high") obtained every 10 min for a 70-min period following the administration of cannabis. The second was a questionnaire administered at the end of each experimental session. The questionnaire data are presented here, while the self-rating data are presented in Chapter 14.

REVIEW OF PROCEDURES

Twenty subjects each smoked five different cannabis preparations on five separate occasions (Chapter 3). The cannabis preparations are listed in Table 3-1. To elicit the subjective experiences during and after smoking, a questionnaire was constructed including those items identified as usual reactions to hashish. The questionnaire was administered at the end of each experimental session, i.e., 70 min after smoking. The items are listed in Table 10-1.

The subjects were asked to answer with yes or no; if the answer was yes, elaboration of the experience was requested. The subjects were also asked about distortions in perception or ideas of persecution; how many drachmas (the monetary unit in Greece) they would have been willing to pay for what they had smoked; and to rate their subjective feelings of *mastura*. Overt

TABLE 10-1. *Reported experiences by subjects during different smoking conditions*

Question	No. of positive answers ($N = 20$)				
	Placebo	Marijuana (78 mg[a])	Hashish (90 mg[a])	Liquid THC-Δ-9 (100 mg[a])	Hashish (180 mg[a])
Did you feel mixed up or confused?	2	6	3	4	2
Did you feel anxious or fearful?	0	4	1	1	3
Did you have any strange or unusual thoughts?	0	8	2	1	4
Did you feel worried or depressed?	6	7	2	0	7
Did you feel happy?	3	16	18	19	15
Did you enjoy smoking?	4	17	18	20	16
Did you feel free and without problems?	5	14	19	19	14

[a]Amount of THC-Δ-9 in the sample.

changes in behavior observed during each smoking session were also recorded.

RESULTS

The experiences reported by the subjects during the various smoking conditions are presented in Table 10-1. The maximum number of responses to those questions that indicated a negative tone (questions 1–4) occurred in the marijuana condition, followed by hashish (180 mg). The responses to the question of confusion indicated that the subjects interpreted it to mean drowsy rather than "mixed-up." One subject smoking marijuana (78 mg) showed a panic reaction and was unwilling to continue the experiment. One subject smoking marijuana (78 mg) saw deformed bodies and thought that the environment was different, with various colors around the room. He also heard "voices" 10–20 min after the end of smoking.

After smoking hashish (180 mg), three subjects became pale; two of them were dysarthric for some time and vomited soon after smoking. After THC-Δ-9 (100 mg), three subjects developed untoward effects; one had auditory hallucinations, and another vomited and became temporarily dysarthric.

The maximum number of "yes" responses to the questions that indicated pleasant tones (questions 5–7) was obtained in the THC-Δ-9 (100 mg) condition followed by hashish (90 mg). Most subjects enjoyed and felt happy with smoking active substances despite the fact that they reported unpleasant experiences. After smoking placebo, the men felt rather depressed and disappointed.

Subjects discriminated all active substances from placebo. Evaluating in drachmas the price they were willing to pay for what they had smoked, the prices given for the four active preparations were significantly higher than for placebo.

DISCUSSION

The cannabis preparations used for these experiments were high in THC-Δ-9 equivalents, and more pronounced adverse reactions were expected (4,81,86,181). During the initial phase of the study (Chapter 5) subjects reported their current use of hashish to be 2.32 times/day, and 3.13 g at each use. During a later experimental phase (Chapter 16), when permitted *ad libitum* smoking, subjects consumed the equivalent of 50–70 mg THC-Δ-9 during each of two smoking sessions. This may be taken as representative of their typical daily consumption and is similar to that which subjects report they consume in present use (3.1 g × 4.5% THC-Δ-9). Yet even with the greater than usual doses noted above, the behavioral reactions to cannabis were minimal, short-lived, and occurred in only a few individuals. Confusion, fragmented thinking, or aggressive behavior were not seen, and every subject cooperated satisfactorily.

We did not assess changes in thought processes by the administration of a specific test, as was done by others. Melges et al. (124) reported temporal disorganization and delusional-like ideation during marijuana intoxication using the "goal directed serial alternation" (GDSA) task. Subjects were given a number between 106 and 114 and were asked to subtract 7; add 1, 2, or 3; and then repeat this alternate subtraction and addition until an exact goal between 46 and 54 was reached. The authors noted a dose-related decrement in temporal disintegration. In attempting to reach the specified goal, subjects frequently lost track of where they were in the serial process. Melges suggests that temporal disintegration has implications for speech construction. Meaningful speech requires that words and phrases be hierarchically ordered in a goal-directed fashion. Indeed, loose associations and lack of goal-directedness in the speech patterns of subjects were identified. Our clinical assessment might not be sensitive in detecting small thought process abnormalities, and these may have been missed. All subjects reported that they were thinking more efficiently than usual, and they expressed feelings of superiority after smoking active materials. These feelings have been described by others (119,191). The absence of acute toxic reactions may be related to the lack of fear of arrest or disruption of family and occupational endeavor. The only subject who developed a panic reaction to marijuana was calmed down quickly after gentle and authoritative reassurance that nothing was seriously wrong. Such modification in behavior reflects the importance of environmental influences in determining the effects of cannabis smoking.

The one subject who developed hallucinations with persecutory delusions after hashish (180 mg) and THC-Δ-9 (100 mg) was not accustomed to high doses. Although the strength of the dose is a factor in these reactions, the role of idiosyncratic variables cannot be overlooked.

These subjects exhibited a clear-cut differentiation of the active cannabis preparations from the placebo. This has not been demonstrated by others (91). In Jones' studies (91) dosage was low and the failure of subjects to separate active drug may reflect dosage and the relative lack of sophistication of the occasional, short-term users assessed in his studies. Volavka et al. (193) demonstrated a clear-cut differentiation in responses to active preparations as compared with placebo in a similar short-term, irregular, American user population when THC-Δ-9 doses were 15–22 mg.

11

Acute Effects of Cannabis on Cognitive, Perceptual, and Motor Performance in Chronic Hashish Users

Rhea Dornbush and Anna Kokkevi

Many tasks have been used to assess cognitive, perceptual, and motor effects of marijuana consumption. Their diversity, as well as the differences in procedure, samples, and experimental conditions, has led to seemingly inconsistent reports of the changes in these functions (29,103,117,143).

The most consistent changes are in time sense and short-term memory, and these measures are most frequently included in batteries of mental functioning. Although subjects report that time passes slowly, the effect has been difficult to demonstrate experimentally using the conventional methods of measurement. These include *reproduction* (the subject is asked to reproduce a time period which was previously indicated); *estimation* (the subject is asked to estimate the length of a given time period); and *production* (the subject is asked to define a period of time). These methods yield different data (12).

Reproduction is the easiest method and requires the subject to count during an interval to be reproduced. No matter what his counting, he merely has to repeat it. Reproduction is insensitive to cannabis effects (51,84). Karniol et al. (95) and Tinklenberg et al. (187) found the production task to result in underjudgments; Jones and Stone (94) did not.

In contrast to the underestimates of time when a production method is used, estimation methods should result in overjudgments. Clark et al. (33) and Jones and Stone (94) obtained overestimations; Weil et al. (200) did not. The outcome of time sense measures varied with the interval used. Shorter intervals, as seconds, are generally overjudged; longer intervals varying from 1 sec to 5 min are underjudged (48,51,188). Further, time sense measures differ when the intervals are filled or empty and when instructions emphasize subjective or objective time (12).

The effects of marijuana on memory are more consistent. Subjects report that they cannot remember the beginning of a sentence or the word immediately preceding the one they are speaking. Among the most sensitive tests of memory change are those involving a delay of recall, even as short as seconds (50,51). These tests permit a more precise definition of the locus of marijuana effects in the memory process. Recall is always near perfect, if not perfect, when it is immediate, i.e., when the item must be repeated without a delay or interpolated task. From this it is assumed that perception, registration, and retrieval of the item is correct. These processes are not affected by marijuana. On the other hand, when a delay occurs between item presentation and recall, retention falls off and a deficit ensues. The interval between presentation and recall is the time when the item must be stored or coded for later retrieval. It is therefore assumed that marijuana affects storage processes (1,42,50,51). A simple digit span, which is an immediate recall task and in which there is minimal involvement of storage processes, is usually not sensitive to marijuana effects (124).

Other categories of mental functioning have not been as extensively or consistently explored as time sense and memory. There is little uniformity in test selection from one study to another; no two studies have used the same methodological procedures. For example, Weil et al. (200) measured sustained attention with a continuous performance task (CPT), alertness using the digit symbol substitution test (DSST), and muscular coordination employing a pursuit rotor apparatus. Caldwell et al. (25) measured auditory and visual acuity and sensory thresholds. The LeDain Commission (111) examined short-term serial position memory and general alertness (DSST). Meyer et al. (129) measured field dependence, attention, alertness, time perception, task focusing, and muscular coordination. Hosko et al. (84) measured reaction time and time sense using the method of reproduction. Jones and Stone (94) measured field dependence with rod and frame apparatus, time sense using methods of estimation and production, and general alertness with DSST. Kiplinger et al. (102) examined motor performance, delayed auditory feedback, and stability of stance, while Barratt et al. (9) examined sleep EEG effects, reaction time, visual closure, and pursuit rotor performance.

In each study a smoking route of administration was used. Others have used an oral route, including Hollister and Gillespie (82), Melges et al. (124), Tinklenberg et al. (189), Waskow et al. (198), and Darley et al. (42).

In addition to the type and route of administration, cannabis effects are also related to time of testing, type of cannabis preparation, characteristics of the user, set, and setting. However, when differences in experimental procedures are evaluated, a general pattern of marijuana effect emerges. The effects of marijuana on cognitive, perceptual, and motor functions are temporary. Complex tasks—those which require simultaneous and coordinated mental operations such as the GDSA or serial sevens, or memory tasks with a delayed recall or multisignal reaction time—are more consistently affected than simple tasks, e.g., digit span or single-signal reaction time or time reproduction tasks (29,124,155). Performance impairment is related to dose: Complex tasks are usually affected by high doses and are less or not at all affected by low doses (12,111).

To assess mental functioning in chronic hashish users in Greece, we selected tests that were similar to those used on American populations and which were as free of cultural limitations as possible. These tests, which sampled the functions of memory, alertness, time sense, mental coordination, and motor performance, included:

1. *Digit span, forward and backward:*[1] This is a subtest of the Wechsler Adult Intelligence Scale (WAIS) and was administered as specified in the WAIS. The subject is asked to repeat ascending lengths of digits both forward and backward. The maximum length is 9.

2. *Barrage de signe:* This is an alertness task, similar to the DSST. Subjects are given a sheet with rows of symbols. Three symbols at the top of the page serve as standards. Subjects are required to cross out the symbols on the sheet that are the same as the three standards. There is a 3-min limit on this task. The score is the number right minus the number wrong.

3. *Time estimation:* Subjects are required to estimate the length of time of the *barrage de signe* task, i.e., 3 min.

4. *Serial sevens:* The subject is given a number and is required to subtract seven from that number until he reaches a designated goal. The time to complete the task and number of errors are combined to yield a fault index.

5. *Star tracing:* The test consists of a six-point star approximately 20 cm in diameter and formed with dots. The subject is asked to draw the star by following the dots, as quickly as possible, without lifting the pencil or turning the paper around. Two scores are obtained: the time required for completion of the test and the errors or number of dots excluded by the line drawn by the subject.

REVIEW OF PROCEDURES

Twenty subjects were used. These subjects were a subsample of the total experimental group of users (Chapter 3). The doses administered are listed in Table 3-1.

The postsmoking evaluation was approximately 90 min in duration. The EEG, heart rate, mood, and other continuously measured variables were assessed for the first 30 min and again from 60 to 70 min. Psychological tests were presented twice: 30–50 min postsmoking and again at 70–90 min postsmoking. Performance during each time period was assessed separately. No statistical comparison of changes in performance between the two time periods was performed.

Data were analyzed by multiple linear stepwise regression, comparing the drugs as a group and each drug separately against placebo. If the main effect of the drug was significant, *post hoc* *t*-tests were performed among the various substances.

---

[1] Despite the fact that this test is usually not sensitive to marijuana effects in American users, we included it in this battery to observe the differences and similarities in performance between American short-term users and Greek long-term users.

Of the five psychological tests presented, three resulted in significant drug effects at one or both time points. Figures 11-1 through 11-5 show performance in these five tests as a function of the quantity of THC-Δ-9 smoked. Table 11-1 shows the means and standard deviations of performance on each of the tests, the *p* values for the drug effect, and the comparisons among drugs that were significant.

Differences Between Placebo and Active Substances

In the *barrage de signe* task, at 30 min all drug conditions except THC-Δ-9 (100 mg) result in impaired performance. Only hashish (180 mg) and marijuana (78 mg) are significantly different than placebo. At 70 min, hashish (180 mg) is still significantly worse than placebo.

All active drug preparations at 30 min, except THC-Δ-9 (100 mg), in the time estimation task result in overestimations of the 3-min task. THC-Δ-9 (100 mg) results in a mean exact estimate of the task, and placebo results in an underestimation. Only hashish (180 mg) and marijuana (78 mg) are different from placebo. At 70 min the same pattern of under- and overestimation are observed as at 30 min. However, the differences are not significant.

In the serial sevens task at 30 minutes, performance is impaired in the hashish (180 mg) condition compared to placebo. At 70 min, however, this difference is no longer significant. No difference in the digit span and star tracing tasks are observed compared to placebo at either 30 or 70 min.

Differences Among the Active Substances

In the *barrage de signe* task at 30 and 70 min, performance is better in the THC-Δ-9 (100 mg) condition than it is under the other three active preparations. In time estimation at 30 min, hashish (180 mg) results in greater overestimation of time than THC-Δ-9 (100 mg). This difference disappears at 70 min.

In serial sevens at 30 min, hashish (180 mg) performance is significantly impaired compared to hashish (90 mg). This difference is not present at 70 min. There are no significant differences among the active substances in the digit span and star tracing tasks at either 30 or 70 min.

Although no statistical comparisons were undertaken between the two time points, performance always improves during the second testing period, especially in the placebo condition (Figs. 11-1 through 11-5). This suggests that improvement reflects an interaction of practice effect and a lessening effect of the drug with time.

DISCUSSION

We found no simple dose-response relationship for cannabis substances in the tasks in which there was a drug effect. Hashish (180 mg), with the largest

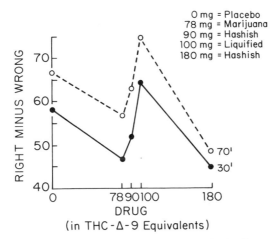

FIG. 11-1. *Barrage de Signe.* Mean correct performance in the *Barrage de Signe* task as a function of quantity of THC-Δ-9 smoked. Data are displayed separately for the two testing periods, 30 min after smoking and 70 min after smoking.

quantity of THC-Δ-9, usually resulted in the greatest impairment, but differences in performance were most prominent and most frequent not only with hashish (180 mg) but also with marijuana (78 mg). Hashish (180 mg) was significantly different from placebo in *barrage de signe,* time estimation, and serial sevens. Marijuana (78 mg) was significantly different from placebo in *barrage de signe* and time estimation. Why hashish (90 mg) and THC-Δ-9 (100 mg), conditions that both contained greater THC-Δ-9 quantities than marijuana, are not different from placebo is difficult to explain. It may be that hashish (90 mg) was most similar to the dose and quality of material

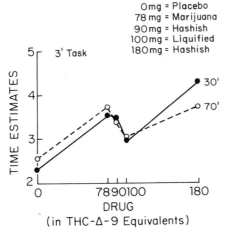

FIG. 11-2. Time estimation. Mean time estimates of a 3-min task as a function of quantity of THC-Δ-9 smoked. Data are displayed separately for the two testing periods, 30 min after smoking and 70 min after smoking.

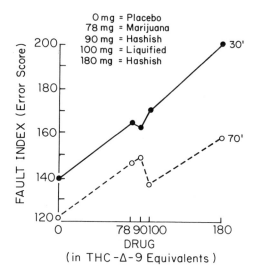

FIG. 11-3. Serial sevens. Mean error (time to complete task × number of errors) score as a function of quantity of THC-Δ-9 smoked. Data are displayed separately for the two testing periods, 30 min after smoking and 70 min after smoking.

that subjects typically used. Marijuana (78 mg), although containing only 12 mg less THC-Δ-9 than hashish (90 mg), had a different combination of cannabinoids. Assays of American marijuana and Greek hashish indicated that marijuana contained less cannabidiol and cannabinol than hashish (Chapter 12).

Recent evidence indicates that different combinations of cannabinoids

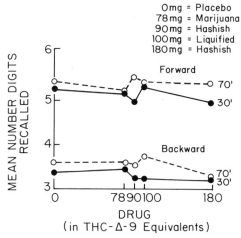

FIG. 11-4. Digit span. Mean number of digits recalled in both forward and backward spans as a function of quantity of THC-Δ-9 smoked. Data are displayed separately for the two testing periods, 30 min after smoking and 70 min after smoking.

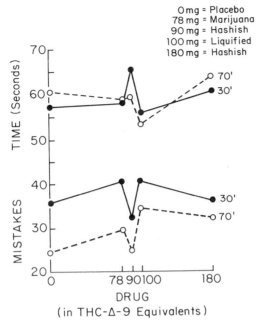

FIG. 11-5. Star tracing. Mean time to complete the star and mean number of dots excluded (mistakes) as a function of quantity of THC-Δ-9 smoked. Data are displayed separately for the two testing periods, 30 min after smoking and 70 min after smoking.

may result in different effects. Karniol et al. (95) found that THC-Δ-9 caused a deficit in time estimation; the effect was blocked when THC-Δ-9 and cannabidiol were consumed together. Therefore marijuana may represent a qualitatively different and new substance for Greek subjects.

The data from the THC-Δ-9 condition are more complex. In the *barrage de signe* condition, performance is actually better than placebo. There are two possible explanations for this result. (a) THC-Δ-9 has a short shelf life; it is affected by light and air and deteriorates rapidly. However, studies of heart rate (Chapter 15) indicate that THC-Δ-9 is as potent as the other cannabis products and results in heart rate increases as great as those produced by hashish (180 mg), the largest dose we administered. (b) It was noted in the methods section that the order of drug presentation was only semirandom. THC-Δ-9 was always the last drug presented, whereas the order of the other drugs was randomized. In the *barrage de signe* task there was a clear order or practice effect (Fig. 11-6). When each drug was the first to be administered, performance was poorest; performance improved steadily as the drug was administered on the second, third, and fourth day of the series. Thus superior performance in the THC-Δ-9 condition may be a result of its order of testing, i.e., always the last day. This suggests a practice effect. That a practice effect was possible under these large doses is itself noteworthy.

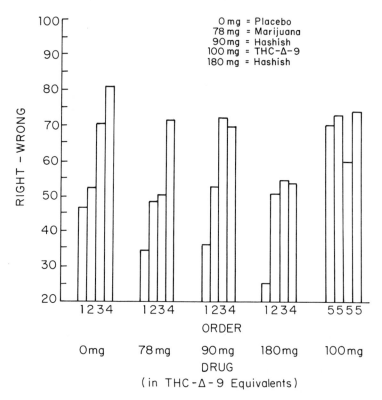

FIG. 11-6. Mean correct performance in the *Barrage de Signe* task as a function of the order of each drug's administration: (1) represents the occasion when the drug was first administered; (2) indicates that the substance was presented on the second day preceded by a different substance (quantity of THC-Δ-9). Order or practice effects occur within the 0, 78, and 90 mg doses and less so with the 180 mg dose, suggesting more of a drug effect at the higher dose.

The time estimation data correlate with anecdotal reports. Users indicate that time passes slowly. To be consistent with these reports, experimental methods of estimation should result in overestimations, as did occur. Under nondrug conditions, time sense is usually underestimated as was the case with placebo. Within this framework, then, a mean exact estimate of the task (i.e., 3 min), which was found in the THC condition, may also be considered a deviation from what would be expected under nondrug conditions.

Greek subjects, after an average of 25 years of cannabis use, evidence a pattern of response on these tests of mental functioning after doses ranging from 78 to 180 mg of THC-Δ-9 which is similar to that of American short-term users consuming up to 25 mg THC-Δ-9; i.e., performance on simple tasks such as digit span and star tracing is unaffected. Performance on more complex tasks (e.g., *barrage de signe,* serial sevens, and time estimation) is affected. The heavy, long-term use of cannabis does not qualitatively change

TABLE 11-1. *Five tests of mental performance as a function of dose (THC-Δ-9 quantity smoked)*

Task	Time	Drug effect** (p values)	Placebo	78 mg Marijuana	90 mg Hashish	100 mg THC-Δ-9	180 mg Hashish	Drug comparisons* .01	Drug comparisons* .05
Barrage de signe	30	0.01	58.05 ± 23.51	46.25 ± 23.13	51.85 ± 27.43	64.16 ± 25.40	44.35 ± 25.94	180 < 100 78 < 100	180 < 0 78 < 0 90 < 100
	70	0.01	66.95 ± 22.15	56.45 ± 23.80	62.85 ± 28.72	74.95 ± 24.97	48.10 ± 23.37	180 < 0 180 < 100 180 < 90 90 < 100 78 < 100	
Time estimation	30	0.05	2.50 ± 2.18	3.55 ± 1.80	3.48 ± 1.85	3.00 ± 1.81	4.30 ± 2.32	180 > 0	78 > 0 180 > 100
	70	n.s.	2.58 ± 2.06	3.70 ± 1.37	3.40 ± 1.91	3.00 ± 1.82	3.75 ± 2.52		
Serial sevens	30	0.05	139.70 ± 64.55	165.76 ± 73.62	163.60 ± 71.78	171.68 ± 73.12	201.50 ± 85.53	180 > 0	180 > 90
	70	n.s.	121.20 ± 69.20	146.80 ± 62.73	148.55 ± 64.18	137.89 ± 63.24	158.30 ± 81.88		
Digit span Forward	30	n.s.	5.30 ± 0.95	5.20 ± 0.93	4.95 ± 1.07	5.32 ± 0.80	5.00 ± 0.84		
	70	n.s.	5.45 ± 0.92	5.20 ± 1.12	5.55 ± 1.07	5.42 ± 0.88	5.40 ± 0.80		
Backward	30	n.s.	3.40 ± 1.07	3.45 ± 0.97	3.25 ± 0.89	3.21 ± 0.89	3.05 ± 0.92		
	70	n.s.	3.60 ± 0.86	3.60 ± 1.02	3.55 ± 0.86	3.74 ± 0.64	3.30 ± 0.90		
Star tracing Time	30	n.s.	57.30 ± 20.30	58.05 ± 20.68	65.65 ± 24.44	50.00 ± 21.54	60.85 ± 21.42		
	70	n.s.	60.45 ± 20.73	58.90 ± 19.80	59.25 ± 18.96	53.16 ± 18.05	64.35 ± 34.44		
Mistakes	30	n.s.	35.35 ± 21.74	40.50 ± 24.15	32.20 ± 16.35	40.26 ± 21.43	36.10 ± 20.02		
	70	n.s.	24.60 ± 15.35	29.40 ± 17.49	24.60 ± 25.15	34.05 ± 18.07	32.15 ± 15.90		

*Comparisons between individual drugs that were significant at p ≤ .01 or p ≤ .05.
**This is the effect of drugs, as a group, compared to placebo.

the patterns of response in acute use exhibited by as-yet occasional, short-term users.

SUMMARY

The more complex tests of mental functioning were adversely affected by certain doses of THC-Δ-9. These effects in all but one instance were short-lived and no longer present 70 min after smoking 180 mg THC-Δ-9 (hashish). This dose also adversely affected *barrage de signe* (this disruption was still present 70 min after smoking), time estimation, and the serial sevens task. Marijuana (78 mg) adversely affected performance in the *barrage de signe* and time estimation task; this has been related to the possibility that marijuana is a qualitatively different substance than the hashish usually smoked by these men. Performance was no different than placebo with 90 or 100 mg THC-Δ-9.

Unexpected was the superior performance in the *barrage de signe* task with the 100 mg THC-Δ-9 (liquified) preparation. Performance was significantly better after 100 mg THC-Δ-9 than after 78, 90, and 180 mg. We attributed this to the order of drug administration—100 mg was the last condition; the other conditions were fully randomized. This suggests a practice effect, which is noteworthy in view of the high doses of cannabis administered. Further evidence of practice effects with high doses of THC-Δ-9 occurs in the withdrawal experiments (Chapter 18).

12

Acute EEG Effects of Cannabis Preparations in Long-Term Hashish Users

Jan Volavka, Max Fink, and C. P. Panayiotopoulos

Replicable EEG effects after smoking cannabis substances have been described for "social," short-term (several years) marijuana users in the United States. The effects consist mainly of a decrease in the average EEG frequency, an increase in the amount of alpha activity, and a decrease in the amount of beta activity (63,80,162,163,193,194). Other EEG effects have also been reported, but these await replication (4,43,94,130,205).

With increasing public concern over the long-term effects of marijuana use, several studies of repeated cannabis administration under controlled conditions were done. Dornbush et al. (51) administered marijuana daily for 21 days to five young American users. The repeated EEG measurements revealed progressive changes in the postsmoking records suggestive of tolerance development or boredom (no control subjects were used).

Tolerance to some (but not all) EEG effects of marijuana was demonstrated in rats in a study of extremely high doses (20 mg/kg) of THC-Δ-9 (150). As quantitative data on the acute EEG effects of cannabis in long-term, heavy users were not available, such information was one of the goals of the study in Athens. We were particularly interested in the following questions: Does cannabis affect the same EEG variables in chronic users as in short-term users? Is the direction of the change the same? Are the effects linearly related to the dose of THC-Δ-9 contained in various preparations? Does chronic use of cannabis result in tolerance to the acute EEG effects of this substance? What is the relationship between the EEG effects on the one hand and other physiological effects on the other?

METHODS

The procedures selected for the acute experiment in Athens were largely comparable to those used in our previous work in New York (54, 55,56,193,194). These procedures are outlined in Chapter 3. Briefly, the baseline EEG was recorded for 10 min before the subjects started smoking. The smoking took approximately 15 min, and no EEG was taken during that period because the subjects were moving as they smoked. After they stopped smoking, the EEG was recorded for 30 min. The recording was interrupted for 20 min, after which another 20-min EEG record was taken.

Twenty subjects were examined, and each had five sessions. The THC-Δ-9 content of the different substances used at each session were marijuana (78 mg), pure THC-Δ-9 (100 mg), hashish (90 and 180 mg), and placebo. The order of administration of the substances, except THC-Δ-9 (100 mg) was randomized. THC-Δ-9 (100 mg) arrived late in Athens and was administered at the last session.

During the EEG the subjects were supine, with their eyes closed. An alerting procedure was used; the subjects were instructed to keep a button depressed, and whenever the button was released a buzzer sounded. The international 10-20 system was used for the EEG electrode placement. Grass P 511 preamplifiers were used. The EEG was recorded on paper and magnetic tape. The tapes were processed at the EEG laboratory of the Department of Psychiatry, State University of New York (SUNY) in Stony Brook. The EEG from the right occipital-vertex derivation was subjected to computerized period analysis. This derivation was selected to maintain comparability with our previous cannabis studies (193,194). A variable Krohn-Hite filter (model 3750 R, slope 24 db per octave) was interposed between the analog tape and the A/D converter to suppress frequencies below 1.1 and above 35 c/s. Relative amounts (percent-time) were computed for four frequency bands: theta (3.5–7.5 c/s); alpha (7.5–13.5 c/s); beta-1 (13.5–18.5 c/s); and beta-2 (18.5–24.5 c/s). In addition, the mean EEG frequency was computed. For these five EEG variables, averages were computed for 10-min segments. Each EEG variable was thus represented by one presmoking and five postsmoking means, which were the data subjected to subsequent statistical analyses.

Hierarchical multiple regression analyses were used. The order in which the variables were entered into the regression equations was determined by the investigators and used to render the regression analyses comparable to analysis of covariance (35). A more detailed explanation of the application of these analyses was presented elsewhere (194,195).

RESULTS

The results of the analyses can be described in terms of differences between the placebo and each of the active substances and differences among the active substances.

Differences Between Placebo and Active Substances

Each of the four active substances decreased the *average EEG frequency* (Fig. 12-1). The decrease ranged between 0.3 and 0.6 c/s. This effect reached its maximum within 20 min after smoking, and it was significant for each

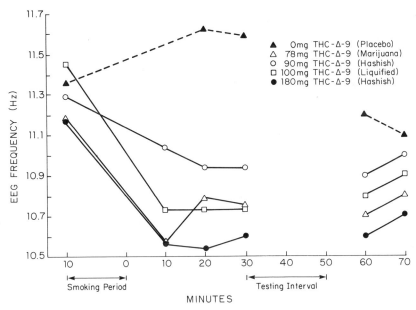

FIG. 12-1. Average EEG frequency (Hz) displayed over time as a function of quantity of THC-Δ-9 smoked.

active preparation during the first 30 min after smoking (Table 12-1). At 60 min the effect of low-dose hashish dropped below the level of statistical significance. No preparation affected the average EEG frequency at 70 min after smoking.

There was an increase of the amount of *theta activity* during the first 30 min after smoking THC-Δ-9 (Fig. 12-2; Table 12-1). The active preparations as a group had an effect on theta activity between 20 and 70 min after smoking. At 20 and 30 min the active preparations tended to increase the amount of theta activity (more so than placebo). At 60 and 70 min THC-Δ-9 elicited more theta activity than placebo; the other three preparations had an opposite effect. In case of high-dose hashish and marijuana, this difference from placebo became statistically significant at 70 min. (The direction of differences from placebo can be inferred from the signs of partial correlation coefficients in Table 12-1.)

The amount of *alpha activity* increased during the first 10 min after smoking each substance, including placebo (Fig. 12-3). The high dose of hashish and also marijuana elicited significantly more alpha activity than placebo; this effect seemed to increase with time after smoking (rather than decrease, as most other effects did). At 60 and 70 min there was a significant group effect (i.e., an effect of the active preparations as a group) showing an increase of the amount of alpha activity (Table 12-1).

All cannabis preparations elicited a decrease of beta activity (Figs. 12-4 and

TABLE 12-1. Comparison between the EEG effects of four cannabis preparations and placebo

	10 min		20 min		30 min		60 min		70 min	
Variables	r_p	F	r_p	F	r_p	F	r_p	F	r_p	F
Average frequency										
THC-Δ-9 (100 mg)	-.53	28.84[a]	-.59	39.94[a]	-.57	35.95[a]	-.56	10.92[a]	-.13	1.25
Hashish (90 mg)	-.32	8.49[a]	-.44	18.84[a]	-.42	15.95[a]	-.21	3.60	-.01	0.01
Hashish (180 mg)	-.52	28.22[a]	-.59	40.01[a]	-.55	32.10[a]	-.37	11.90[a]	-.16	1.95
Marijuana (78 mg)	-.52	28.34[a]	-.48	22.00[a]	-.47	21.84[a]	-.29	7.13[a]	-.10	0.69
"Drug group"		11.15[a]		13.72[a]		11.78[a]		3.99[a]		0.74
Theta										
THC-Δ-9 (100 mg)	.23	4.25[b]	.29	6.77[b]	.34	9.72[a]	.17	2.13	.01	0.01
Hashish (90 mg)	.11	0.92	.18	2.49	.11	0.99	-.03	0.09	-.18	2.38
Hashish (180 mg)	.01	0.01	.07	0.34	.03	0.08	-.13	1.27	-.26	5.27[b]
Marijuana (78 mg)	.03	0.07	-.02	0.03	-.01	0.01	-.18	2.45	-.30	7.61[a]
"Drug group"		1.52		2.81[b]		3.75[a]		2.88[b]		3.57[b]
Alpha										
THC-Δ-9 (100 mg)	.00	0.00	.07	0.36	-.01	0.01	.09	0.58	.22	3.85
Hashish (90 mg)	.06	0.28	.09	0.64	.11	0.92	.16	1.95	.26	5.48[b]
Hashish (180 mg)	.24	4.77[b]	.19	2.96	.22	3.98[b]	.29	6.69[b]	.38	12.38[a]
Marijuana (78 mg)	.24	4.62[b]	.25	5.13[b]	.21	3.36	.33	9.04[a]	.43	16.71[a]
"Drug group"		2.30		1.51		1.93		3.27[b]		5.09[a]
Beta-1										
THC-Δ-9 (100 mg)	-.52	29.23[a]	-.55	32.48[a]	-.50	25.57[a]	-.39	13.58[a]	-.38	12.72[a]
Hashish (90 mg)	-.32	8.55[a]	-.43	17.14[a]	-.39	13.44[a]	-.30	7.52[a]	-.28	6.37[b]
Hashish (180 mg)	-.53	29.05[a]	-.55	33.03[a]	-.47	21.11[a]	-.38	13.04[a]	-.37	11.59[a]
Marijuana (78 mg)	-.55	32.91[a]	-.51	26.73[a]	-.45	18.65[a]	-.39	13.70[a]	-.44	17.65[a]
"Drug group"		12.44[a]		11.64[a]		8.54[a]		5.07[a]		5.39[a]

TABLE 12-1. (Continued)

	Partial correlation coefficients and F ratios at 10–70 min after smoking									
	10 min		20 min		30 min		60 min		70 min	
Variables	r_p	F	r_p	F	r_p	F	r_p	F	r_p	F
Beta-2										
THC-Δ-9 (100 mg)	−.30	7.16[a]	−.49	24.26[a]	−.43	17.39[a]	−.33	9.09[a]	−.30	7.40[a]
Hashish (90 mg)	−.24	4.48[b]	−.39	13.52[a]	−.34	9.55[b]	−.23	4.09[b]	−.21	3.55
Hashish (180 mg)	−.40	14.49[a]	−.51	26.68[a]	−.46	19.88[a]	−.39	13.37[a]	−.33	9.03[a]
Marijuana (78 mg)	−.39	13.81[a]	−.48	22.77[a]	−.44	17.99[a]	−.40	14.54[a]	−.34	9.90[a]
"Drug group"		4.84[a]		9.28[a]		7.12[a]		4.89[a]		3.20[b]

The entries summarize the results of 25 multiple regression analyses; i.e., a separate analysis was used to examine the difference between each of the five EEG effects of a placebo preparation and four cannabis preparations at each of five points in time after the preparation was smoked. In each analysis the EEG measure was the dependent variable. The independent variables, listed in order of entry in the regression equation, were *subjects* (as dummy-coded variables), *the presmoking EEG effect*, and the cannabis preparations (dummy-coded with placebo as the reference variable). Thus the effects of intersubject differences and the presmoking EEG levels were accounted for prior to investigating the drug effects. The results of analyzing the covariates (*subjects* and *presmoking EEG*) are not presented. Instead, the table provides the partial correlation coefficients (r_p) and F ratios associated with each of the cannabis preparations. Each r_p indexes the relationship of the dichotomous variable which represents its associated cannabis preparation and placebo to the dependent variable after all other cannabis-placebo comparisons have been taken into account. The statistical significance of the relationship is indexed by the F ratio associated with it. In the present experiment a significant r_p may be interpreted to mean that the EEG effect of its associated cannabis preparation is different from that of placebo. The independent variable called "drug group" refers to the significance of the amount of EEG variance that can be attributed to the set of four cannabis preparations. The statistical degrees of freedom for the individual drug effects is (1, 75); for the "Drug group" effects it is (4,75).

[a]p ⩽ .01.
[b]p ⩽ .05.

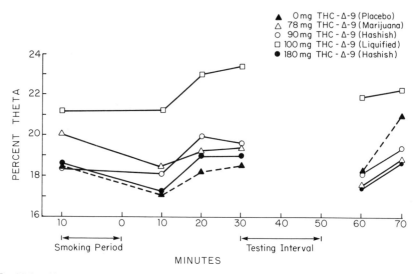

FIG. 12-2. Mean percent theta activity displayed over time as a function of quantity of THC-Δ-9 smoked.

12-5). The decrease started within the first 10 min after smoking and lasted for 70 min. The depression of beta activity was significant during each 10-min segment for each cannabis preparation, except for low-dose hashish at 70 min (Table 12-1). Beta-1 and beta-2 bands behaved very similarly.

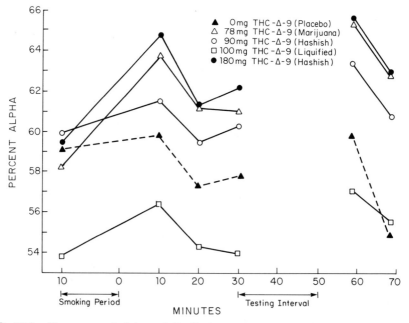

FIG. 12-3. Mean percent alpha activity displayed over time as a function of quantity of THC-Δ-9 smoked.

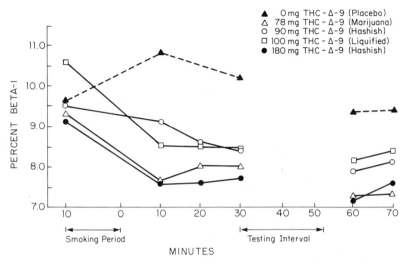

FIG. 12-4. Mean percent beta-1 activity displayed over time as a function of quantity of THC-Δ-9 smoked.

Differences Among the Active Substances

When the drug group effect was significant, *post hoc t*-tests were used to explore the differences among the active substances. Table 12-1 indicates that the drug group effect was significant in 20 regression analyses. Six pairs were constructed from the four drugs, and the significance of the difference between the members of each pair was tested. This made a total of 120 *t*-tests (20 × 6). Eighteen of these *t*-tests yielded significant differences.

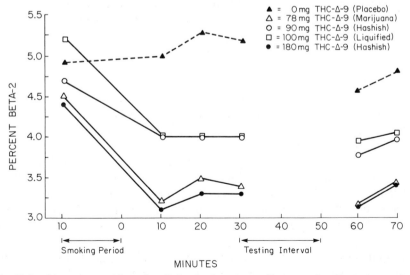

FIG. 12-5. Mean percent beta-2 activity displayed over time as a function of quantity of THC-Δ-9 smoked.

The tests comparing THC-Δ-9 with the other drugs gave significant differences more frequently than those comparing marijuana and the two doses of hashish with each other. Of the 18 significant results, 13 tests were those involving THC-Δ-9.

THC-Δ-9 decreased the *average EEG frequency* more than the low-dose hashish during the first 30 min after smoking (Fig. 12-1). It increased the amount of *theta activity* more than the other three active substances did at 20–30 min after smoking. All substances were associated with some increase of the amount of theta activity at 70 min; THC-Δ-9 showed a significantly smaller increase than either high-dose hashish or marijuana (Fig. 12-2). THC-Δ-9 elicited a significantly smaller amount of *alpha activity* at 60 and 70 min than marijuana (Fig. 12-3). It depressed *beta-1* activity more than the low-dose hashish did (Fig. 12-4).

Only five tests yielding significant differences failed to involve THC-Δ-9. Three of these five tests confirmed that 180 mg THC-Δ-9 (hashish) had a greater effect than 90 mg THC-Δ-9 (hashish) on the average EEG frequency and on the amount of beta-1 activity. Marijuana (78 mg THC-Δ-9) had more effect than low-dose hashish (90 mg THC-Δ-9) on the same EEG variables.

DISCUSSION

The three cannabis substances elicited the same pattern of EEG activity in the long-term users—a pattern of activity similar to that observed in U.S. occasional users of cannabis smoking smaller doses (10–22.5 mg THC-Δ-9 equivalent) in either single doses or daily administration for 21 days (50,55,57,58,162,163,193,194). The increase in alpha activity, the slowing of the mean alpha frequency, and the decrease in beta activity were the principal measured effects in the U.S. users. In addition, changes occurred in the theta frequency band which had not been observed in the U.S. population. The general pattern of EEG effects was similar across cannabis preparations, doses, and populations.

However, there are differences in the relative activity among the cannabis preparations studied. We believe the variations in the Greek and U.S. studies to be partly due to the different compositions of these substances. In addition, in the Greek studies the experimental design may have contributed to the differences in activity of the substances.

Table 12-2 summarizes the contents of cigarettes smoked in single doses. High- and low-dose hashish and marijuana were assayed to contain 180, 90, and 78 mg THC-Δ-9 per dose, respectively. THC-Δ-9 has been considered to be the principal (if not the only) compound responsible for the physiological and psychological effects of cannabis. Our results, however, cannot be explained as exclusive effects of THC-Δ-9.

Assuming that the THC-Δ-9 elicits essentially all cannabis effects, it might be predicted that the two active drugs to show the maximal difference from

TABLE 12-2. *One-dose contents of substances used*

Substance	THC-Δ-9 (mg)	Cannabinol (mg)	Cannabidiol (mg)
Hashish (4 g)	180	66	74
Hashish (2 g)	90	33	37
Marijuana (3 g)	78	12	3
THC-Δ-9	100	0	0

Data are based on the NIMH assays of materials we used.

each other would be high-dose hashish ($\cong$ 180 mg THC-Δ-9) and marijuana ($\cong$ 78 mg THC-Δ-9), since the difference in the THC-Δ-9 content per dose is the greatest for the active substances. This expectation is not supported, however: Of 18 significant differences among the four active substances, none occurred between high-dose hashish and marijuana. This could mean that substances other than THC-Δ-9 had important effects. We have data from cannabinol (CBN) and cannabidiol (CBD) assays (Table 12-2). Assuming that these two substances are active, one would expect the maximum of differences to occur between pure THC-Δ-9 and the other three active substances. This expectation is supported: Of 18 significant differences among the active drugs, 13 tests involved THC-Δ-9.

Karniol et al. (95) found CBD to interfere with the effects of THC-Δ-9 on pulse rate and mood in man. More recently, Dalton et al. (41) found that combining CBD (150 μg/kg) with THC (25 μg/kg) significantly attenuated the subjective euphoria of THC-Δ-9 in male volunteers, while CBD alone was inactive. In another experiment, CBD smoked 30 min before THC-Δ-9 did not affect the THC-Δ-9 response, indicating that CBD effects were short-lived. If CBD were to interfere with the EEG effects of THC-Δ-9 in our experiment, the substances containing CBD should show less effect than expected on the basis of their THC-Δ-9 content. Conversely, pure THC-Δ-9 should show relatively more effect because its action was not impeded by CBD. Our data support this prediction. High-dose hashish showed less effect on theta activity than the pure THC-Δ-9 in spite of the fact that it contained much more THC-Δ-9 per dose than the pure THC-Δ-9 cigarettes. This applied to the measurements taken at 20 and 30 min after smoking; at 70 min the hashish exerted a more powerful effect than the pure THC-Δ-9, indicating that the interaction effect persisted for 30 min. A similar inversion of theta effect direction also occurred at 70 min after marijuana.

At 60 and 70 min THC-Δ-9 elicited a significantly smaller amount of alpha activity than marijuana. This last difference is perhaps related to the subjective effects of pure THC-Δ-9. Our experiments in U.S. users revealed that as far as the pleasantness of the smoking experience is concerned, 20 mg THC-Δ-9 was not different from placebo. Hashish and marijuana cigarettes, each calibrated to contain 20 mg THC-Δ-9, were perceived as significantly more pleasant than placebo. Karniol et al. (95) reported that "CBD in all doses used, was able to partially block this anxiety component of THC-Δ-9 action, leaving the subjects less tense and enjoying the experiments more." The differential effects of THC-Δ-9 on subjective feeling (*mastura*) is discussed elsewhere in this volume (Chapter 14). We can assume that the 100 mg pure THC-Δ-9 elicited some anxiety, which in turn interfered with the increase of alpha activity. The amount of alpha activity in the waking adult generally decreases with anxiety and increases with relaxation.

Our experimental procedures with the Greek long-term users also may have contributed to the observed differences between the THC-Δ-9 preparations and the other substances. As mentioned earlier, pure THC-Δ-9 was the only substance administered in a nonrandom order (always at the last session). The starting (presmoking) levels of alpha activity were somewhat lower for the THC-Δ-9 than for the other sessions (Fig. 12-3); the opposite seems to be true for the beta and theta activities, suggesting that a sequence effect was present. We did account statistically for the variance contributed by the presmoking EEG levels but were unable to account for the sequence effect in THC-Δ-9 sessions.

Assuming that CBD interfered with the action of THC-Δ-9 in hashish, one would hypothesize that the marijuana (containing 78 mg THC-Δ-9 and 3 mg CBD per dose) activity would be proportionally greater and the decrement due to CBD less. Our data support such a hypothesis. Marijuana elicited a significantly larger decrease of the average EEG frequency and of the amount of beta-1 activity than the low-dose hashish. Both these differences were observed during the first 10 min after smoking.

The finding that the effects of marijuana were greater than those expected on the basis of the THC-Δ-9 content is open to an alternative explanation. This was the first time our Greek subjects were exposed to American marijuana. It is possible that it contained some unidentified active compounds. Would these compounds potentiate the THC-Δ-9 or have additive effects? If these compounds were absent from the Middle Eastern hashish that the Greeks had customarily used, they would not have been tolerant to them. Consequently the response to these compounds would contribute to the total effect of marijuana. These unidentified compounds are of course strictly hypothetical; we have no evidence of their existence. Our data support the observations that the physiological effects of THC-Δ-9 are decreased by other compound(s) present in the native substances, and CBD is one likely candidate for such interfering activity.

In these studies also, Greek long-term hashish users smoked doses of 78–180 mg equivalent THC-Δ-9 with physiological effects that were similar to the much lower doses (10–22.5 mg) used in U.S. experimental studies. In our dose-finding experiments in long-term users, we observed their smoking lower doses of cannabis substances, and in each instance they reported these lower doses to be of minimal or limited activity. Although we failed to undertake a systematic dose-tolerance study, we believe the observations that these men smoked these large doses without untoward effects—without the toxicity reported by Tassinari et al. (185) or Hollister (81) using lower doses—to be indicative of the development of tolerance. In our 21-day inhalation studies in U.S. subjects, we believe we observed the onset of tolerance in the reduced increase in heart rate and in the percent of alpha activity enhanced with successive doses (50). In recent reports Cohen (36), Jones and Benowitz (93), and Mendelson (125) present equally compelling data regarding the development of tolerance to successive doses of cannabis if exposure is repeated for at least 7–21 days.

SUMMARY

Long-term cannabis users smoked placebo, marijuana, hashish, and THC-Δ-9-impregnated material in a laboratory setting. The THC content of the active substances was assayed as 78 mg for marijuana, 90 mg and 180 mg for the two doses of hashish, and 100 mg for the THC-Δ-9. Sessions were randomized for four substances; the THC-Δ-9 was the last substance in each subject.

The principal EEG effects of the active substances were an increase in the amount of alpha activity, a decrease in the mean alpha frequency, a decrease in beta activity, and a biphasic effect on theta activity. These effects were similar for all substances, and different from placebo. The degree and duration of the effects increased with the amount of THC and decreased with the amount of CBD in the smoked material. The high doses smoked by these men without severe toxicity were interpreted as a manifestation of tolerance to cannabis.

13

Visual Evoked Responses in Chronic Hashish Users

C. P. Panayiotopoulos and Costas Stefanis

The human brain's electrical responses to sensory stimulation (evoked responses) have been used to study the effect of many drugs on the electrocortical activity in man. The results from a small number of studies on the effect of THC-Δ-9 on evoked responses are conflicting. This may be attributable to differences in stimulus parameters, recording techniques, dose, and subject characteristics, including chronicity in the use of THC-Δ-9.

Rodin et al. (162,163) examined 10 male freshmen medical students who admitted to long-term use of marijuana. All had used other "psychedelic" drugs (mescaline, LSD, psilocybin). Evoked response averaging for 15 head locations was carried out for three different sensory modalities, i.e., light, sound, and passive joint movements. The recordings were made before smoking and after the subjects had reported the presence of their usual "high." During each session two to three cigarettes were smoked *ad libitum* so that each subject smoked 1.2–11.7 mg THC-Δ-9. Rodin et al. (162,163) did not find consistent changes in the average evoked responses at these doses, with any stimulus.

After oral administration of THC-Δ-9 (0.35 mg/kg), Tinklenberg et al. (188) found both latency and amplitude changes in visual response components evoked by patterned light stimulation. Latencies were prolonged, and the amplitudes of a late negative (200 msec) and positive (280 msec) waves were increased.

Lewis et al. (113) studied an "occasional user" group (marijuana was not used more than twice per month for the preceding 3–4 years) and a "frequent user" group (marijuana was used twice or more weekly for 3–4 years). Subjects were tested on five occasions in a randomized sequence with the first session on a control session. Subjects ingested placebo and THC-Δ-9 (0.2, 0.4, and 0.6 mg/kg) contained in sugar. Unipolar recordings were obtained from O_1, O_2, C_3, C_4, F_3, and F_4 electrodes. Visual (VER) and somatosensory evoked responses were recorded 2, 3, and 4 hr after ingestion. With the exception of the positive wave occurring at 110 msec, the occipital VER components were increased in latency ($p < 0.05$) by the largest doses of THC-Δ-9 (0.6 mg/kg). The VERs from the other locations

(C_3, F_3) were also late (to a lesser extent) when the subjects smoked THC-Δ-9 (0.6 mg/kg). The N_2–P_3 component recorded from O_1 was attenuated ($p < 0.05$) by all dose levels. No differences in latency in somatosensory responses were found. The time between THC-Δ-9 ingestion and the recording of evoked responses (2, 3, and 4 hr after drug administration) had little effect on latency or amplitude of the evoked response.

Tassinari et al. (185) reported that high single doses of THC-Δ-9 (0.7–1.0 mg/kg) administered orally in normal volunteers increased the amplitude of the late (after 200 msec) rhythmic VER component.

METHOD

In the present study the effect of varying doses of THC-Δ-9 on VERs of chronic hashish smokers was examined. The drugs administered are described in Table 3-1.

The VERs were studied in the first 12 subjects of the total group of 20. VERs were recorded 25 min before smoking and 45 min after the end of smoking. O_2–C_4 bipolar derivation (stick-on silver-silver chloride electrodes) were used for VER recording. The technique is detailed in Panayiotopoulos et al. (140).

Each flash was delivered every 2 sec through a Beckmann 5561 photostimulator (flash duration 10 μsec, intensity 750 candle-power). The lamp was placed 30 cm in front of the subject's open eyes; the subject was instructed to look at the center of the lamp.

Fifty responses were averaged. The amplitude of the various components was measured as shown in Fig. 13-1, i.e., from the peak of the measured

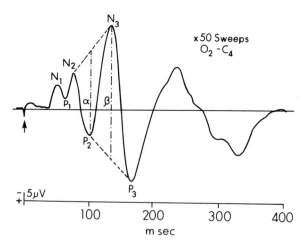

FIG. 13-1. Method of amplitude measurement of visual evoked response (VER) components.

TABLE 13-1. *Effect of THC-Δ-9 on visual evoked responses (N = 12)*

Component	0 mg Pre	0 mg Post	78 mg Pre	78 mg Post	90 mg Pre	90 mg Post	100 mg Pre	100 mg Post	180 mg Pre	180 mg Post
					LATENCY (msec)					
P_1	73.6 ± 9.6	76.0 ± 8.5	76.0 ± 11.8	75.9 ± 11.5	73.8 ± 11.7	78.3 ± 11.2	74.9 ± 11.3	73.9 ± 10.7	75.8 ± 9.7	75.5 ± 7.6
N_2	88.5 ± 10.4	91.6 ± 9.2	88.6 ± 11.3	91.3 ± 14.8	87.3 ± 11.9	90.6 ± 11.3	86.7 ± 12.0	90.7 ± 13.9	88.8 ± 10.7	91.0 ± 11.5
P_2	114.5 ± 7.6	116.7 ± 8.9	114.8 ± 8.4	118.1 ± 8.5	113.6 ± 7.5	115.1 ± 8.5	111.1 ± 11.2	115.8 ± 9.6	111.8 ± 10.7	115.8 ± 8.5
N_3	150.5 ± 14.6	158.3 ± 16.6	155.3 ± 16.4	158.3 ± 17.2	154.3 ± 16.3	156.1 ± 16.9	154.8 ± 9.3	157.1 ± 12.9	156.0 ± 13.3	159.3 ± 17.6
					AMPLITUDE (μV)					
P_1	4.7 ± 2.7	4.7 ± 2.8	4.0 ± 2.6	5.2 ± 2.2	4.1 ± 2.2	4.9 ± 2.5	5.2 ± 3.0	5.2 ± 2.5	4.3 ± 1.8	4.5 ± 2.4
N_2	12.1 ± 7.3	12.0 ± 8.2	9.9 ± 6.6	10.7 ± 6.2	10.6 ± 7.1	11.8 ± 8.7	9.3 ± 6.2	12.3 ± 8.0	10.2 ± 5.8	12.2 ± 8.0
P_2	20.5 ± 13.0	20.7 ± 12.0	22.5 ± 12.2	24.2 ± 14.2	21.5 ± 12.5	24.5 ± 16.1	18.5 ± 11.0	20.4 ± 11.4	20.5 ± 12.2	25.6 ± 13.7
N_3	29.8 ± 14.7	27.0 ± 13.7	30.4 ± 14.3	36.0 ± 17.3	27.4 ± 12.1	35.8 ± 14.4	27.8 ± 15.3	33.1 ± 20.3	27.6 ± 14.8	37.6 ± 22.0

Results are given as the mean ± SD.

93

component to the point at which a vertical line crosses another line which joins the peaks of the preceding and following VER components.

Multiple, stepwise linear regression analyses were used to examine the drug effects on the eight VER variables (amplitude P_1, N_2, P_2, N_3, and latency P_1, N_2, P_2, and N_3). A detailed description of the analyses is in Chapter 12. Both the subject variance and presmoking VERs are removed prior to evaluating the effect of drugs of postsmoking values.

RESULTS

Table 13-1 shows the means and standard deviations for the eight VER variables. In testing the contribution of the drug set to the variance of the VER measures, we found amplitude N_3 to be significantly increased ($F = 4.64$; df 4,40, $p \leq .01$). *Post hoc* t-tests between drugs indicate that the N_3 amplitude after THC-Δ-9 (100 mg) was lower than after hashish (180 mg) and hashish (90 mg). In 10 of 12 chronic hashish smokers, the N_3 wave increased after smoking hashish (180 mg). No differences were found in the latency of the VER components.

DISCUSSION

The changes in VER following smoking high doses of cannabis by long-term hashish users were small, being limited to an increase in amplitude of a late VER component. Although no confident comparisons can be made between our results and those reported by others, it is interesting that Tinklenberg et al. (188) and Tassinari et al. (185) also found an increase in the amplitude of the late component.

Animal studies suggest that the principal sites of action of THC-Δ-9 are probably cerebral association areas and their related subcortical structures (19,46,47). The present results (i.e., that THC-Δ-9 does not affect the early VER complex) are compatible with the above view.

The positive VER components have been related to inhibitory postsynaptic potentials, whereas the negative VER components have been related to excitatory postsynaptic potentials (39). The finding that THC-Δ-9 increases the amplitude of negative (N_3) late VER components might indicate a stimulant effect of THC-Δ-9.

14

Intercorrelations Between Physiological and Psychological Effects of Marijuana, Hashish, and THC-Δ-9 in Long-Term Hashish Users

Peter Crown, Rhea Dornbush, and Jan Volavka

The increase in heart rate and the subjective feeling of being "high" are two of the most frequently reported responses to acute cannabis administration. THC-Δ-9 is an active principle of cannabis that is at least partly responsible for both these effects. A heart rate increase related to the dose of THC-Δ-9 has been reported by a number of observers (2,81,129,160, 194,195).

The subjective effects of cannabis are usually monitored by self-reporting scales based on the descriptive nouns employed by cannabis users (e.g., "high," "stoned") to describe the intoxicated state (164). The magnitude of the subjective effect has been related to the ingested dose of THC-Δ-9 and the increase in heart rate (64,86,195). Although there does appear to be a "high" factor (111), work in our laboratory demonstrated that the experience is not uniformly pleasant. While the "high" was found to increase linearly with heart rate, "pleasantness" followed an inverted U relationship, increasing with the heart rate up to 102 beats/min and then decreasing with higher heart rates (193).

The physiological and psychological effects of long-term cannabis use have been investigated in experimental populations and in populations with a history of long-term daily hashish use. When cannabis was administered daily for several weeks, the heart rate increase following smoking generally diminished with time (15,50,61). This diminution in the heart rate response occurs as early as the fifth day of smoking (50). A decrease in the heart rate response has also been observed despite an increase in dosage. Mendelson et al. (127) noted that subjects who smoked marijuana *ad libitum* for 21 days increased their consumption by 37–46% from the first to the last 5 days of the study, but the size of the heart rate response still diminished over this period.

The subjective effects ("high") with repeated smoking have been less consistent. In a study conducted in our laboratory, subjects smoked marijuana (14 mg THC-Δ-9) for 21 days (50). Four of the five subjects reported intense and persistent subjective effects during the first 7–10 days, followed by a decrease and leveling off to the end of the experiment. Rossi et al. (164) reported a similar diminution in the "high" in their 21-day *ad libitum* study, but this change did not reach statistical significance. Each day the subjects rated themselves as significantly "higher" after the last smoking of the day compared to the first smoking of the day. Williams et al. (205) also found a gradual increase in the number of marijuana cigarettes smoked daily over a 39-day period, but both heart rate increase and the "high" disappeared after the first few days.

In the present study of long-term users of hashish, the relations between self-ratings of "high," drug type, dose, and heart rate are assessed.

REVIEW OF METHODS

Twenty subjects were studied, each participating in five sessions. The doses administered are listed in Table 3-1. A 10-min presmoking baseline EEG and electrocardiogram (ECG) were recorded; the ECG was also recorded during the 15-min smoking period. The postsmoking period was approximately 90 min in duration. The EEG and ECG were recorded continuously for the first 30 min and again from 50 to 70 min. Heart rate was determined from the ECG. For a review of EEG procedures, see Chapter 12.

Means were computed for 10-min intervals for heart rate and EEG. Thus there was one presmoking mean, one during-smoking mean for heart rate only, and five postsmoking means at 10, 20, 30, 60, and 70 min.

Mastura (a Greek word combining the qualities of the English words "high" and pleasant) was a self-rating, measured on a scale of 1–10, with 10 being the "highest and best ever." *Mastura* ratings were obtained every 10 min (i.e., at 10, 20, 30, 60, and 70 min) to correspond with EEG and heart rate measures.

At the end of the first 30 min subjects were asked how many drachmas (the monetary unit in Greece) they would have been willing to pay for what they had smoked. This was an open-ended measure.

Multiple linear stepwise regressions were used to evaluate these data (35). This technique is similar to analysis of covariance. It permits the investigator to determine the order of entry of the independent variables into the regression equation. In all analyses, effects of intersubject variance were accounted for prior to investigating any other relationships. Separate analyses were performed for each 10-min measurement.

These analyses compared: (a) the drugs as a group against placebo and (b) the significance of each drug separately against placebo. If the main effect of a drug was significant (defined as $p \leq 0.05$) then *post hoc* *t*-tests were performed to determine differences among the active drugs.

RESULTS

The acute behavioral and EEG effects of the cannabis preparations are detailed in Chapters 10–13. In general, these substances elicited the behavioral effects the men reported from their daily hashish use.

Differences Between Active Drugs and Placebo

Heart rate: The four active drugs, taken as a group, increased heart rate compared to placebo (Fig. 14-1). Each drug considered separately also increased the heart rate more than did the placebo. This increase is observed from the end of the smoking period and continues through the last observation 70 min after smoking.

Mastura: The effects of the active drugs on the *mastura* scale ratings were similar to heart rate effects: higher *mastura* ratings were given following the active drugs compared to placebo (Fig. 14-2). Each active drug compared individually with placebo increased the *mastura* ratings at all time points.

Drachmas: The analyses showed that the active drugs as a group and individually produced higher drachma responses than placebo.

Differences Among Active Drugs

Heart rate: THC-Δ-9 (100 mg) and marijuana (78 mg THC-Δ-9) had consistently greater effects on heart rate than did hashish (90 mg THC-Δ-9).

Mastura: Hashish (180 mg THC-Δ-9) produced higher *mastura* ratings at

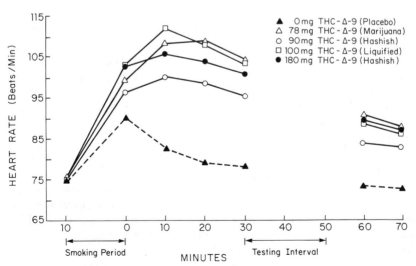

FIG. 14-1. Mean heart-rate response over time as a function of THC-Δ-9 quantity consumed.

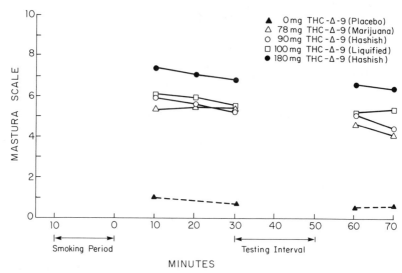

FIG. 14-2. Mean *mastura* (mood) ratings over time as a function of THC-Δ-9 quantity consumed.

all time points than any other drug. There were no other differences among active drugs.

Drachmas: Hashish (180 mg THC-Δ-9) had a greater effect on drachma ratings than did hashish (90 mg THC-Δ-9) and THC-Δ-9 (100 mg).

Relationships Among Variables

Heart rate and mastura: There was a postitive relationship between heart rate and *mastura*. To determine whether this relationship was mediated by the drugs, separate analyses were done in which the drug effects were statistically accounted for prior to determining the relation between heart rate and *mastura*. These analyses find that a portion of the heart rate variance (1–3%) is related to *mastura* independent of drug effects. This was true for the analyses using data from the first, second, and third 10-min segments, as well as for the data at 60 min after smoking.

Heart rate and drachmas: The heart rate observed 30 min after smoking was related to the price subjects said they would be willing to pay for what they had just smoked. However, when the variance contributed by drugs to the drachma response was accounted for, the relationship between heart rate and drachmas was no longer significant, indicating that, unlike HR and *mastura,* the relationship was mediated through the drugs.

EEG and mastura: The acute effects of the cannabis preparations on EEG are detailed in Chapter 12. The present discussion is concerned with the relationship between EEG changes and subjective effects, as measured by the *mastura* scale. Five EEG variables were assessed at 10, 20, 30, 60, and

70 min after smoking. The results indicate that the increase of alpha activity at 70 min after smoking was related to higher *mastura* ratings. Decreases in beta-1 and beta-2 were related to higher *mastura* ratings at all time points, and the decreased mean EEG frequency was related to higher *mastura* ratings at all time points except 70 min. There was no relationship between theta activity and *mastura* ratings. If the variance contributed by the drugs was first accounted for, however, the relationship between EEG and *mastura* scores was no longer significant. Thus the relationships between EEG and *mastura* scores were not independent of the drug effect.

DISCUSSION

Acute cannabis administration in long-term hashish smokers results in an increased heart rate, and the heart rate is directly related to the subjective feelings of being "high" (*mastura*). This relationship exists independently of drug effects. On the other hand, the relationships between EEG and *mastura*, and between drachmas (price) and heart rate, are not independent of the drug effect.

The present data suggest that the THC-Δ-9 content of different cannabis preparations does not exhibit a linear dose-response relationship with heart rate. Marijuana containing 78 mg THC-Δ-9 produced higher heart rates than hashish containing 90 mg THC-Δ-9. This occurred for the duration of the 60-min period after smoking. Also, the greatest mean heart rate was observed 10 min after smoking 100 mg THC-Δ-9. The heart rate at this time was greater than the hashish which contained 180 mg THC-Δ-9. On the other hand, 100 mg THC-Δ-9 produced higher heart rates than hashish containing 90 mg THC-Δ-9.

Previous studies have suggested that there is a positive linear relationship between the THC-Δ-9 content of cannabis and an increased heart rate (81,194). Although such a linear relationship may exist for pure THC-Δ-9 or for similar substances containing different amounts of THC-Δ-9, present results may be due to the fact that the three different types of cannabis preparations (hashish, marijuana, and THC-Δ-9) each contained different proportions of cannabidiol (CBD). Karniol et al. (95) demonstrated that CBD has a blocking effect on pulse rate and subjective effects of THC-Δ-9 in man. In the present study the CBD/THC-Δ-9 ratios were 0.41 for hashish and 0.04 for marijuana, a 10-fold difference in ratio. It is probable that the interaction between CBD and THC-Δ-9 reduced the heart rate response to a greater degree for hashish than for marijuana, and for the same reason 100 mg pure THC-Δ-9 produced the highest mean heart rate of all preparations.

If CBD does block THC-Δ-9 effects on heart rate and the feeling of being "high," why then did hashish containing 180 mg THC-Δ-9 produce the highest *mastura* ratings, given its high CBD content? In our studies of cannabis effects in the United States, we found that although "high" was related linearly to heart rate, the feeling of "pleasantness" followed an inverted U function of heart rate (indeed, other words describing subjective effects may show still other relationships with physiological measures). The word *mastura* was chosen as the scale in Greece because it is in common use, just as the word "high" is used in America. This creates a difficulty in making comparisons because the two seemingly different effects are confounded in one word. Comparisons aside, it may be that the relative proportions of THC-Δ-9 and CBD in hashish account for hashish producing the effect most desired in the Greek population.

The statical analyses indicate that the relation between EEG and *mastura*, and between heart rate and drachmas, can be fully explained by the simultaneous action of drugs on both variables in each pair. Figure 14-3 illustrates the point. The relation between heart rate and *mastura* is different in that it is partly independent of the drug effect. This implication stems from the fact that a significant portion of the heart rate variance is related to *mastura* even if drug effects are accounted for. This finding must be interpreted with caution. The portion of heart rate variance accounted for by *mastura* independently of drugs is very small (1–3%), and its size raises questions about its importance. On the other hand, we did report an analogous relationship in another experiment employing American marijuana users (193).

We do not know whether this finding reflects a causal relationship between heart rate and subjective effects of cannabis. Would the increase of heart rate be the cause or the effect of the "high"? It is perhaps important that in the Athens study the highest heart rate (following 100 mg THC-Δ-9) did *not* correspond with the highest *mastura* rating. Galanter et al. (64) measured the plasma THC-Δ-9 concentrations, pulse rate, and "high" simultaneously. Peak pulse rate coincided with peak plasma THC-Δ-9 levels 5 min after smoking, but the peak "high" occurred approximately 50 min after smoking. At this time heart rate was already decreasing.

Tolerance to cannabis effects is suggested in the present study in the large quantities of THC-Δ-9 tolerated by these subjects as compared with American subjects. The Greek subjects had approximately equivalent heart rate

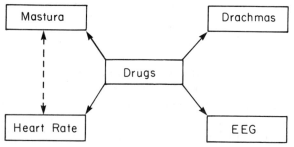

FIG. 14-3. Relationship between drugs and *mastura* (mood), heart-rate, EEG, and drachmas (price willing to pay).

and "high" responses to 180 mg THC-Δ-9 compared with Americans smoking 20 mg THC-Δ-9 (193). If tolerance is defined as "an adaptive state characterized by diminished response to the same quantity of a drug" (52), the question of tolerance in the Greek population could be answered more directly by systematic investigation of their responses to lower doses, as well as those doses currently being investigated.

In spite of the fact that the Greek subjects were accustomed to smoking high doses of hashish for many years, the time course of their responses was similar to that of American users studied in our laboratory. In both groups the peak heart rate was observed 10 min after smoking and was still elevated approximately an hour after smoking, with the "high" (*mastura*) following the same time course.

SUMMARY

The relationships between EEG measures, heart rate, and self-ratings in chronic smokers exposed to experimental doses of hashish, marijuana, and THC-Δ-9 were examined. Heart rate increases were related to self-ratings of "high" and were independent of drug changes in the price subjects were willing to pay for drug; the EEG measures, self-ratings, and price willing to pay, however, were dependent on drug and dose. The heart rate increase was not linearly related to the dose, suggesting a CBD-THC-Δ-9 interaction in hashish and marijuana.

15

Psychophysiological Effects of Acute Cannabis Inhalation

Aris Liakos, John Boulougouris, and Costas Stefanis

Psychophysiological measures have long been used in cannabis research as indices of autonomic changes or of level of arousal with inconsistent results. For example, an increase in heart rate is the most frequently reported index of the effects of cannabis on acute administration. The response is dose-related and closely associated with the THC-Δ-9 content of the cannabis material used (90,102,160). Although the pulse rate increases following smoking, slow pulse rates have also been reported in cannabis users after oral administration (146), and bradycardia may occur hours after the administration of cannabis (92).

The effects on temperature, pupil size, plethysmography, respiration, and galvanic skin response (GSR) are less frequently reported and less well defined. Some authors report a fall in body temperature after cannabis administration (83,86,198), whereas others report no change (85) or even a rise in temperature (205). Early studies of pupillary changes report dilatation of the pupil (3,4,7,147), whereas more recent studies report no change (46,86,147,200) or constriction (77,78).

Lung-irritating effects of cannabis smoking are reported, but changes in respiratory rate are inconsistent (85,86,200), as are the effects on blood flow. Rickles et al. (161) report no change in forearm blood flow, whereas Beaconsfield et al. (10) report an increased blood flow. No changes in GSR were found by Rickles et al. (161), but Low et al. (116) reported a decrease in skin conductance level.

Among the reasons for inconsistent results may be the use of single doses of cannabis. Studies in long-term users at high doses are few, being limited to experimental prolonged marijuana administration (50,60,92). In this chapter the psychophysiological effects of four different cannabis preparations in long-term hashish users are described.

Details of the experimental design are found in Chapter 3. Subjects smoked placebo, marijuana leaf (78 mg THC-Δ-9), and hashish (two doses: 90 and 180 mg THC-Δ-9) in a randomized double-blind design. They also smoked 100 mg THC-Δ-9 infused on placebo on a separate occasion. The materials were mixed with tobacco, as is habitual in long-term users in Greece, and rolled into large cigarettes identical in appearance. Pulse rate, respiration, temperature, pupil size, GSR, and finger pulse volumes were recorded for varying periods before, during, and after smoking.

TECHNIQUES OF MEASUREMENT

Subjects were examined in an individual temperature-controlled room. They were seated in a comfortable chair, and the electrodes were placed. Following a 2-min rest period recording of skin conductance level, a table with a chin rest and lights for pupil measurement were rolled in front of the subject, and the pupil measurement was taken. After a 2-min rest period recording, the first shock was administered and the reaction recorded until the pen returned to the baseline. This was followed by a 2-min rest period recording; and then the second shock was given and the reaction recorded.

Two identical shocks were administered for each subject to assess skin conductance response. To estimate the intensity suitable for each subject, on the first day and before the experiment started a sample of electric shocks of increasing intensity were delivered to the subject until he said that it was unpleasant but that he was able to tolerate it. The mean intensity of shocks used for all 20 subjects was 3.5 milliamperes, and the duration of the shock was 1 sec.

Electrodermal Activity

Two measures reflecting the change in level of arousal were taken: skin conductance level (SCL) and skin conductance response (SCR). They were recorded presmoking and 75 min postsmoking. The device used for measurement utilized the constant-current principle and provided a current output of 70 mV fed into a DC amplifier of a two-channel recorder (Nihon Kohdan, model RM 20). Amplification characteristics of the recording apparatus were such that the sensitivity used gave a 10-mm pen deflection for 30% change of the background level of resistance. The silver chloride electrodes were placed on the distal phalanges of the thumb and third finger. SCR scores were obtained by subtracting the skin conductance level just before electric shock was administered from the maximum deflection in SCL within 3 sec after the stimulus. Scores were converted to square root micromhos before the statistical analysis.

Pulse Rate

The ECG was recorded from two standard ECG electrodes attached across the body—one on the left ankle, the other in the V_4 ECG position. The R wave of each ECG cycle was counted during each 1-min period to provide the true pulse rate for that minute.

Pulse rate was continuously monitored for the presmoking (10 min) and the postsmoking (30 min) periods. There was an interval of 25 min after which a second postsmoking period was recorded (20 min). The analyses were performed on 10-min averages; comparisons are for data at 10, 20, 30, 60, and 70 min.

Finger Pulse Volume

Finger pulse volume (FPV) was measured during the same times as pulse rate. A photoelectric plethysmograph was applied to the subject's left index finger, which was kept in the same position on the arm of a chair during the recording period. The signal for pulse volume was amplified and recorded through a filter on the polygraph so that a deflection of 11 mm corresponded to 0.1 mV. Gains were set the same for all subjects, and measurements were taken every 5 min. The score consisted of the average height (in millimeters) of six consecutive beats.

Respiration

Respiration was monitored through a conventional chest transducer using one channel of the polygraph. One-minute samples of the respiratory rate at 10, 20, 30, 60, and 70 min after smoking were used in the analyses.

Temperature

A thermistor transducer was placed in the left axilla of the subject. A Sanborn 780-8 patient monitor was used with a sensitivity of 0.1°C. Temperatures were registered every 5 min on a recording sheet. Although room temperatures were not rigorously controlled, the room was air-conditioned and heated under control of a room thermostat.

Pupil Size

Color slides were taken with a Pentax SV reflex camera from a distance of 45 cm under standard illumination of two 300-watt bulbs fixed at 1 meter distance and angles of 45° from the head of the subject. Subjects rested on a chin rest. The light was on for 10 sec before the photograph was taken. Slides were projected to a standard maximum horizontal iris diameter of 5 cm, and the maximum horizontal pupil diameter was measured (in millimeters) with a transparent ruler. In cases where the right and left pupil sizes differed, the mean was calculated (114).

Iris size is variable from subject to subject, and a positive relationship between iris and pupil size has been previously demonstrated (60). By expressing pupil size in artificial units characterized as "enlarged pupil," iris size was standardized and part of the intersubject variability was eliminated. Actual pupil diameter (millimeters) was calculated according to the equation $p = (i/I)p$, where p = artificial pupil size (millimeters), i = actual iris size (millimeters), and I = artificial iris size (50 mm). Iris diameter was found to vary between 11 and 12.4 mm (mean 11.7 mm) in a previous study (60). Using this data, (i/I) was calculated to vary from 0.22 to 0.25. This means that our artificial units are approximately four to five times larger than the actual ones. The slides were measured without knowledge of the substance the subjects smoked or the time the measure was made. One presmoking and two postsmoking measurements were obtained (at 30 and 75 min).

DATA PROCESSING

Polygraph data were measured by hand. In the statistical analyses of each measure, a stepwise multiple regression analysis was used. The effect of intersubject variance was accounted for before investigating any other relationships. The drugs as a group and each one separately were contrasted to placebo. If the drug main effect was significant, *post hoc* *t*-tests were performed to determine significant differences between the various drug conditions. The THC-Δ-9 (100 mg) condition was not included in some analyses, as these data were not collected under randomized conditions.

RESULTS
Pulse Rate

As a group and individually, the active drugs significantly increased heart rate compared to placebo (Fig. 14-1, Chapter 14). The heart rate increase is observed from the end of the smoking period and persists to the observation 70 min after smoking.

Finger Pulse Volume

The height of the pulse wave was measured. As a group, drugs differed significantly from placebo at 30 min. The active substances except hashish (90 mg) resulted in a decreased FPV at this time point. *Post hoc* *t*-tests showed no significant differences in FPV between drugs.

Respiration

There were no differences in respiratory rate between the active drugs and placebo (Fig. 15-1).

Temperature

Drugs as a group did not differ from placebo (Fig. 15-2).

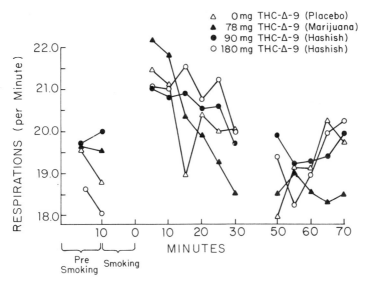

FIG. 15-1. Respiratory rate displayed over time as a function of amount of THC-Δ-9 smoked.

Pupil Size

Enlargement of pupil size was observed at 30 and 75 min after cannabis inhalation (Fig. 15-3). *Post hoc t*-tests showed that THC-Δ-9 (100 mg) and marijuana (78 mg) elicited greater effects than hashish (90 mg) at 30 and 75 min postsmoking. At 75 min postsmoking, the effects of 180 mg THC-Δ-9 (hashish) was also greater than 90 mg THC-Δ-9 (hashish).

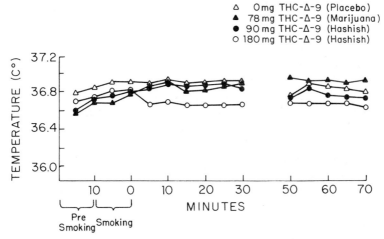

FIG. 15-2. Temperature °C displayed over time as a function of amount of THC-Δ-9 smoked.

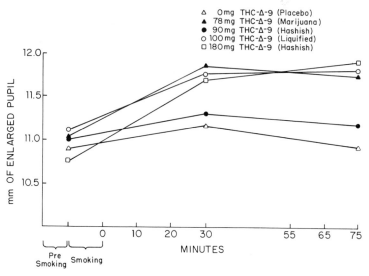

FIG. 15-3. Pupil size displayed over time as a function of amount THC-Δ-9 smoked.

Electrodermal Activity

Skin conductance level was decreased in comparison to placebo 75 min after smoking. There is also a drug group effect (Figs. 15.4 and 15.5).

DISCUSSION

The increase in heart rate, decrease in FPV, and pupillary dilation indicate that inhalation of cannabis is associated with a sympathomimetic release. This arousal is not inhibited in long-term cannabis users, despite their apparent tolerance to cannabis. The doses at which they experience their "high" are sufficient to trigger autonomic effects in addition to the CNS changes. Despite this evidence of sympathetic arousal, subjects experience feelings of relaxation, also seen in the drop in conductance level, increase in EEG alpha activity and decrease in fast beta EEG activity.

As with many previous studies with less experienced users, the tachycardia is related to the THC-Δ-9 content of the material (87,90,102,136,160). The large doses administered to long-term users produced heart rate changes similar to those obtained with much lower cannabis doses in naive and less experienced users in the United States (50,83,193). Although the present study shows a dose-related effect, 180 and 90 mg THC-Δ-9 derived from hashish produced lesser changes than expected for their THC-Δ-9 content. As with the EEG effects, it is probable that interactions between cannabidiol and cannabinol with THC-Δ-9 affected the cardiac response.

The observed decrease in FPV 20–30 min after smoking differs from the increase in blood flow following cannabis reported by Beaconsfield et al.

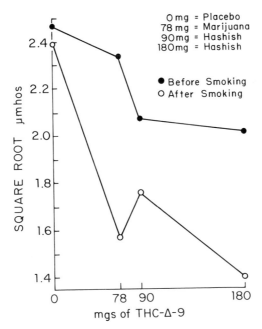

FIG. 15-4. Skin conductance response to first shock measured before smoking and 75 min after smoking as a function of amount of THC-Δ-9 smoked.

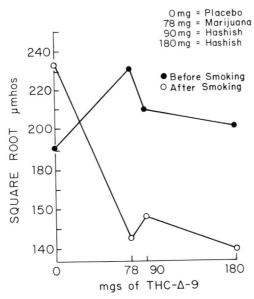

FIG. 15-5. Skin conductance response to second shock measured before smoking and 75 min after smoking as a function of amount THC-Δ-9 smoked.

(10). The difference in observation may be related to population differences, since they used small cannabis doses in naive subjects. The absence of blood flow changes after cannabis reported by others (161) may be explained by the low doses of material used.

The dilation effect on the pupil is consistent with older reports of the effects of cannabis. Most of these reports, however, are noncontrolled descriptions of case histories (3,4,7). Recent controlled pupillary measurements failed to demonstrate pupillary changes (46,47,86,200). In these studies relatively small, single doses of cannabis were used, and the light conditions are not specified. The dilating effects on the pupil in our studies were obtained after high doses of cannabis were administered and under bright illumination.

SUMMARY

Inhalation of diverse cannabis substances by long-term hashish users elicited tachycardia, a decreased finger pulse volume and skin conductance level, and pupillary dilation without changes in the respiratory rate or skin temperature.

ACKNOWLEDGMENT

The editors are grateful to Professor Bernard Tursky of the State University of New York at Stony Brook for assistance in reviewing these findings.

Results: Withdrawal Studies

16

Ad Libitum Consumption and Abstinence

Rhea Dornbush and Max Fink

Most experimental studies of marijuana typically involve standard doses of either smoked or oral material for a single administration or in daily administrations. Doses vary from under 5 mg to usually not more than 25 mg THC-Δ-9 and are administered during a finite smoking period (49–51,83,188,201). Jones (92), however, administered a total daily dose of 210 mg THC-Δ-9 orally at 4-hr intervals for 10–18 days.

Ad libitum smoking studies are considerably less common. This is curious, as there is much anecdotal evidence to suggest that in real-life smoking subjects titrate to inhale quantities sufficient to achieve their subjective "high." In experimental settings, Caldwell et al. (25) and Rodin and Domino (162) permitted *ad libitum* smoking on a single occasion until subjects reached their subjective "high." Caldwell's subjects smoked the equivalent of 6.28 ± 1.2 mg THC-Δ-9, with 300 mg of marijuana in each cigarette; the marijuana was assayed at 1.3% THC-Δ-9. Rodin's subjects consumed the equivalent of 11.31 ± 1.04 mg THC-Δ-9. His cigarettes also contained 300 mg with 1.3% THC-Δ-9 content. The Commission of Inquiry into the Non-Medical Use of Drugs (111) estimated that street use of marijuana in North America varies from 2.5 to 10 mg THC-Δ-9, with an average of 5 mg. Two prior studies of *ad libitum* smoking are noted, and in one the effects of withdrawal were examined. Williams et al. (205) studied *ad libitum* consumption of marijuana. With pyrahexyl, which was orally ingested, daily doses ranged from 60 to 2,400 mg for 26–31 days. Subjects reported the drug to be similar in action to, but stronger than, marijuana. Subjects lost interest in their surroundings, were unable to concentrate on a single item for any length of time, and a few were semistuporous. After 4–6 days the effects decreased; with an increase in dose, effects returned. Abstinence symptoms were present after the second day of nonuse. The marijuana phase was studied for 39 days. Marijuana was smoked and was of unknown potency. Subjects smoked 10–22 cigarettes each day, and there was a gradual increase in the amount smoked each week. With the abrupt cessation of smoking, there were no objective signs of abstinence.

More recently Mendelson et al. (126) permitted subjects to smoke marijuana in any amount and at any time during each 24-hr period for 21 days. Each cigarette contained 1 g of marijuana with a 2.1% THC-Δ-9 content. Subjects were divided into casual-user and heavy-user groups on the basis of previous frequency of use. Casual users averaged two cigarettes a day during the early part of the smoking period and increased gradually to three cigarettes a day by the end of the testing period. Heavy users increased their consumption from four cigarettes a day to more than six and a half cigarettes by the end of the smoking period.

In the present study we examined the effects of the cessation of *ad libitum* smoking of cannabis in long-term hashish users. Subjects smoked both marijuana and placebo, each for 3-day periods, *ad libitum* during specified smoking sessions in a design in which 3 days of smoking cannabis or placebo were followed by smoking the other. In addition, abstinence signs were used to assess the presence of withdrawal symptoms during the 3-day noncannabis smoking period. Several recent studies with repeated administration and abrupt cannabis withdrawal in naive or experienced American users failed to demonstrate physical withdrawal symptoms after *ad libitum* cannabis administration. There is also increasing evidence in the literature to suggest that long-term cannabis users tolerate and consume large amounts of cannabis without severe untoward effects (11,34,166) or abstinence signs.

REVIEW OF PROCEDURES

Subjects smoked twice a day for 6 days. They received placebo cigarettes for 3 days and marijuana for 3 days. Eight subjects received the placebo-marijuana order (order 1), and eight received the marijuana-placebo order (order 2). The start of the second smoking period on each day was 4.5 hr after the start of the first smoking period.

Cigarettes contained 1 g of either active or placebo material. All cigarettes were mixed with tobacco. Active and placebo material was supplied by NIDA. The marijuana had a 2.6% THC-Δ-9 content, and each active cigarette contained 26 mg THC-Δ-9. Placebo was free of cannabinols and cannabinoids.

Subjects were voluntarily admitted to a closed hospital setting for a 6-day testing period. For 2 days prior to hospital admission, they came to the laboratory and smoked marijuana *ad libitum* twice a day. Ready-made cigarettes were available to the subject, and he was instructed to smoke as much as he pleased; the smoking period was 30 min.

RESULTS

The number of placebo and marijuana cigarettes smoked during both smoking periods on each day is shown in Table 16-1 and Fig. 16-1. Two three-way analyses of variance were performed: one on the placebo data and one on the marijuana data. For both analyses, order (placebo to marijuana,

marijuana to placebo), day (1, 2, 3), and smoking period (first period, second period) are the main variables.

Cigarettes Consumed

Marijuana

More marijuana is smoked in order 1, i.e., when smoking follows a 3-day abstinence period (placebo) than when smoking precedes the abstinence period. Furthermore, a greater amount of marijuana is smoked during the first smoking period in order 1 than during the first smoking period in order 2.

Placebo

The mean number of placebo cigarettes smoked decreased significantly during the 3-day testing period. More cigarettes were consumed during the first smoking period than during the second. As was the case with the

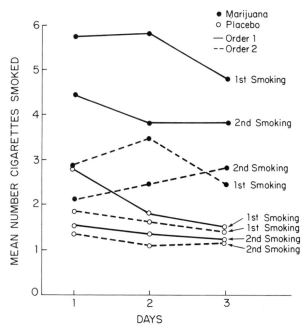

FIG. 16-1. Mean number of marijuana and placebo cigarettes smoked on each day of the experimental period. In order 1 subjects smoked placebo cigarettes for the first 3 days and marijuana for the second 3 days. In order 2 subjects smoked marijuana for the first 3 days and placebo for the second 3 days. There were 2 smoking periods on each day. (Each cigarette contains 26 mg THC-Δ-9).

TABLE 16-1. Number of cigarettes smoked and THC-Δ-9 equivalents

	Day 1	Day 2	Day 3	Day 4	Day 5	Day 6
ORDER 1	PLACEBO			MARIJUANA		
First smoking						
Cigarettes (mean ± SD)	2.72 ± 1.08	1.78 ± 0.92	1.43 ± 1.02	5.65 ± 1.66	5.70 ± 1.52	4.83 ± 0.89
THC-Δ-9 (mean)				146.90	148.20	125.58
Second smoking						
Cigarettes	1.37 ± 0.79	1.09 ± 0.63	1.21 ± 0.52	4.40 ± 1.15	3.76 ± 1.03	3.78 ± 1.15
THC-Δ-9				114.40	97.76	98.28
ORDER 2	MARIJUANA			PLACEBO		
First smoking						
Cigarettes	2.75 ± 0.71	3.50 ± 1.85	2.38 ± 1.19	1.75 ± 1.04	1.63 ± 1.19	1.44 ± 1.12
THC-Δ-9	71.50	91.00	61.88			
Second smoking						
Cigarettes	2.06 ± 0.94	2.38 ± 1.19	2.69 ± 1.16	1.50 ± 0.93	1.38 ± 1.25	1.19 ± 1.16
THC-Δ-9	53.56	61.88	69.94			

marijuana cigarettes, a greater number of placebo cigarettes were smoked during the first smoking session in order 1 than during the first smoking session in order 2.

Smoking Session

The variables measured (i.e., psychological test battery, physiological changes) were recorded each day after the first smoking period. After the second smoking period, psychological performance was measured on the third and sixth days, and physiological variables on the second and fifth days. To permit comparisons between the days in the sequence and the time of day when each variable was measured with the content of the cigarettes smoked prior to the recording period, analyses were performed on the number of cigarettes consumed separately for each smoking session.

First Smoking

A three-way analysis was performed: order, drug, and day in the 3-day sequence are the main variables. All the psychological tests and the physiological and blood pressure measurements recorded after this smoking period are compared using the smoking data of this analysis. More cigarettes were smoked in the first order (5.3) than in the second (2.92) (Fig. 16-2). More marijuana cigarettes were smoked than placebo, and more cigarettes were smoked on the second day, fewer on the first day, and least on the third. Considerably more marijuana was smoked in order 1 than in order 2, whereas the amount of placebo smoked was approximately the same in both order.

Second Smoking

A two-way analysis of variance was performed on the quantities of cigarettes smoked on the second and fifth days. Order and drug were the main variables. The physiological data recorded on days 2 and 5 after this smoking can be compared using the cigarette data of this analysis. More marijuana was smoked than placebo. As was the case with the first smoking session data, more marijuana cigarettes are smoked in order 1 than in order 2 (3.76 and 2.38, respectively) (Fig. 16-3).

A two-way analysis of variance was performed on the quantities of cigarettes smoked on the third and sixth days; order and drug were the main variables. The psychological test data recorded after this smoking on days 3 and 6 can be compared with this analysis. More marijuana cigarettes were smoked than placebo cigarettes. The interaction between order and drug condition that was significant with first and second smoking on days 2 and 5 is not significant here. This is shown in Fig. 16-4. Although the amount of

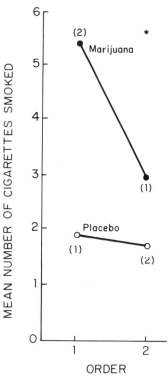

FIG. 16-2. Mean number of marijuana and placebo cigarettes consumed during the first smoking period in each order of drug administration. (1) indicates which substance was administered first in each order; (2) indicates the substance administered second in each order. The asterisk (*) indicates that the interaction between order of drug administration and drug itself is significant.

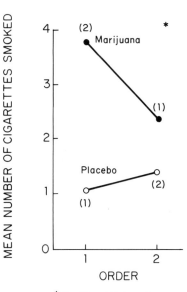

FIG. 16-3. Mean number of marijuana and placebo cigarettes consumed on days 2 and 5 during the second daily smoking period in each order of drug administration. (1) indicates the substance administered first in each order; (2) indicates the substance administered second in each order. The asterisk (*) indicates that the interaction between order of drug administration and drug itself is significant.

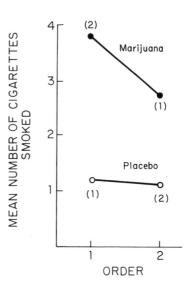

FIG. 16-4. Mean number of marijuana and placebo cigarettes consumed on days 3 and 6 during the second daily smoking period in each order of drug administration. (1) indicates the substance administered first in each order; (2) indicates the substance administered second in each order.

marijuana smoked in order 1 (i.e., after withdrawal) is greater than that smoked in order 2 (i.e., before withdrawal), the difference is not significant.

DISCUSSION

The marijuana smoking data in order 2 (where marijuana precedes abstinence) may be taken as an index of the typical daily consumption of these users (Chapter 5). These men reported an average number of times of smoking each day as 2.32, consuming an average of 3.13 g hashish. During the first and second smoking periods in this study, the men used 50–70 mg THC-Δ-9 (except during one session when they smoked 91 mg).

These men smoked a greater number of cigarettes in the placebo-marijuana order than the marijuana-placebo order, and in each instance smoked less the second smoking each day than the first. Within each order there is a decrease in the amount smoked on each of the 3 days. Furthermore, the men consumed a greater amount of cannabis material after a period of abstinence than when they had an adequate amount of drug available.

There is one measure of cannabis effect that parallels these observations. In this study heart rate was measured 4 hr after smoking. The heart rate increase at this time was greatest on day 1 in each order and decreased rapidly to placebo levels on day 3 (Fig. 16-5). The self ratings of *mastura* immediately after smoking are higher when smoking marijuana in order 1 (placebo-marijuana) than in order 2 (marijuana-placebo). On the other hand, self-ratings are generally higher after the second smoking than after the first smoking (Fig. 16-6). Fewer cigarettes were smoked during the second session (3.1) than during the first (4.1). This suggests that quantities consumed

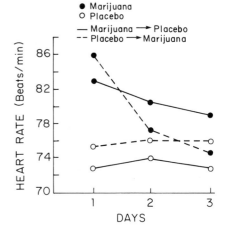

FIG. 16-5. Heart rate response recorded 4 hr after the first daily smoking session.

during the first and second sessions may be additive for *mastura* ratings. During the second daily session subjects may smoke less because they are still experiencing the subjective effects (the "high") from the first smoking.

These observations suggest that some effort at replacing a deficiency or achieving a certain behavioral state requires a greater degree of cannabis inhalation after a withdrawal period. However, satiation to these effects occurs rapidly, not only in the self-ratings but in the heart rate as well.

Whether the increase in the amount of marijuana consumed after a forced abstinence period (order 1) represents a physiological or a psychological response is unclear. A 3-day abstinence period is probably not long enough to deplete the amount of THC-Δ-9 in the body, since the half-life of THC-Δ-9

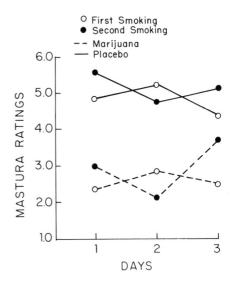

FIG. 16-6. *Mastura* ratings recorded immediately after the first and second daily smoking periods.

is 28 hr in the blood of chronic users and 57 hr in nonusers (112). It is likely that THC-Δ-9 is metabolized more rapidly in chronic users, although its distribution in tissues is the same for both groups (112,145). The drug and its metabolites probably accumulate in tissues when administered repeatedly and are released slowly, as THC-Δ-9 appears in urine and feces for at least 7 days after smoking (112). It is difficult to use these biochemical data alone to explain our findings, for it is also possible that in chronic users THC-Δ-9 may be metabolized more rapidly and the tissues are in fact depleted within a 3-day period. Depletion of THC-Δ-9 may explain the increased smoking seen on day 1 in the men who had the abstinence period.

Alternatively, the tissues may have a build-up of materials ordinarily blocked by THC-Δ-9, and in the absence of this substance the subjects experience the dysphoria of withdrawal and so smoke more to increase the tissue buildup. This interpretation is similar to that suggested for opiate withdrawal symptoms (88). In either case, the greater amount of cannabis consumed after a period of abstinence indicates that there is a process in chronic users which sustains the continued use of cannabis—a process that underlies physiological dependence to cannabis.

It is also probable that the first smoking is adequate to satisfy most of the needs of these men, with the second smoking largely redundant. They smoked less during the second daily session, evinced a lesser heart rate response from this smoking, but valued it more (suggesting an additive effect which may be specific to subjective effects). These observations indicate that the duration of action of cannabis on inhalation is considerably longer in chronic users than the studies in short-term users would indicate.

The absence of withdrawal phenomena reflected on the investigated parameters is consistent with the failure of other systematic studies to demonstrate withdrawal symptoms after repeated cannabis administration and abrupt cessation (50,61,127). They are at variance with Jones and Benowitz (93) who reported a number of withdrawal symptoms after repeated administration of high doses of marijuana in experienced users, and various clinical reports of abstinence symptoms in smokers (14,22). Jones' subjects orally ingested the material and were unable to control the dosage, as is the case with *ad libitum* smoking administration. The presence of symptoms may have been induced by the schedule of administration, which is similar to a prescription schedule and is not typical of the manner or timing of use in social situations.

17

Withdrawal from Cannabis: Psychological Test Performance

Rhea Dornbush and Anna Kokkevi

Tolerance after repeated THC-Δ-9 administration has been demonstrated in rats, dogs, pigeons, and chimpanzees (53,123). Grilly et al. (67) found that a single administration of THC-Δ-9 disrupted performance in a delayed matching-to-sample task in chimpanzees. With repeated THC-Δ-9 administration, the drug effect was reduced.

McMillan et al. (123) found that reinforcement schedule-controlled behavior in pigeons was disrupted by a single administration of THC-Δ-9. With repeated administration, however, the disruptive effects of THC-Δ-9 on schedule behavior disappeared even when the dose was increased to 20 times its original level. Nontolerant pigeons given the increased dose died. Abrupt discontinuation of THC-Δ-9 administration in tolerant pigeons had no effect on their response rate. The same results were obtained with rats.

In other studies Ford and McMillan (59) demonstrated that pigeons continued to work for food after receiving 6,000–18,000 times the minimally effective dose of THC-Δ-9. Abrupt withdrawal of THC-Δ-9 in monkeys was followed by a well-defined autonomic and behavioral abstinence syndrome (96,97).

There are few systematic studies of tolerance to, and withdrawal from, THC-Δ-9 in man. Particularly lacking are estimates of the effects of psychological test performance in long-term users (203). Williams et al. (205) conducted a six-subject study with pyrahexyl compound (judged qualitatively similar to marijuana) and a six-subject study using marijuana. Subjects smoked marijuana *ad libitum* for 39 days preceded and followed by 7 days of nonsmoking observation. In tests of various mental and psychomotor functions, comprehension and analytical thinking were made more difficult; in tests that required concentration and manual dexterity, there was an increase in speed but a decrease in accuracy. Transient "jitteriness" followed abrupt cessation of smoking.

The National Commission on Marijuana and Drug Abuse (134) conducted studies on marijuana acquisition for a 21-day smoking period in 10 heavy and 10 casual users. The subjects were observed as inpatients. Generally, no impairment of performance on tests of cognitive and motor functioning were observed prior to, during, or following marijuana smoking. Rather, there was an improvement in memory and psychomotor performance with time, consistent with the "practice effect." Memory was assessed by digit-span performance, a test in which improvement normally occurs on repeat testing. The same is also true for the psychomotor task, a "shooting gallery" event. Other tests included the Halstead Category test, tactical performance test, Seashore Rhythm test, finger tapping tests, and trail making tests. Practice effects occurred where expected. Tolerance did seem to develop, but it did not follow classic definitions of the phenomenon. Some users smoked up to 200 mg THC-Δ-9 during a daily administration (obviously implying tolerance), but they did not require these large doses for an effect.

In the Canadian Commission study (111) the longest smoking period was 52 consecutive days. Subjects worked for tokens which in turn were traded for desired objects, including additional marijuana. Subjects were confined during observation. Under mandatory drug conditions, subjects were increased from 16 to 30 mg THC-Δ-9. However, when there were no mandatory doses and subjects were permitted free purchase, they smoked 2–4 mg THC-Δ-9. The mandatory large doses were subjectively unpleasant. During free-purchase periods, marijuana intake did not increase with time. Initially, subjects who smoked the smaller doses evidenced greater work productivity than those who received mandatory high doses. Tolerance to this effect may have occurred during the course of the experiment. At the end of the smoking period, differences in work productivity were minimal. There was no evidence of a withdrawal syndrome or signs of dependence.

Dornbush et al. (50) administered marijuana to users for 21 consecutive days. The test period was preceded and followed by drug-free periods. THC-Δ-9 (14 mg) was administered in a single dose. Assessments included tests of short-term memory and the digit-symbol substitution test (DSST). After an initial decrement, there was an improvement in short-term memory; the DSST improved without an initial decrement. Because there was no control group, it was difficult to attribute improvements in performance to either practice or to tolerance. The study does show, however, that marijuana does not inhibit a subject's ability to improve with practice, i.e., exhibit positive transfer. All subjects reported a sense of well-being and euphoria. However, there was a decrease in subjective effects during successive sessions, with the greatest changes occurring after the first week. This "tolerance" to subjective effects also has been reported in other chronic studies (134).

Frank et al. (60) conducted a daily administration study in healthy users who were hospitalized for the duration of the study. They smoked 7 mg marijuana (with either 1% or 2% THC-Δ-9) for 28 consecutive days, preceded and followed by nonsmoking periods. There was no evidence of cumulative effects, withdrawal, or tolerance in psychological parameters.

Perez-Reyes et al. (145) administered an intravenous infusion of THC-Δ-9 on a single occasion to a group of infrequent marijuana smokers (less than one cigarette per month) and a group of frequent users (several times per day for at least the preceding year). If tolerance or sensitivity to active components of marijuana had developed, frequent users would have responded differently than infrequent users to THC-Δ-9. There were no differences between the two groups, however, in the amount of THC-Δ-9 needed for a perceived effect, to accelerate heart rate, in the total dose administered, or in the maximum level of the "high." The distribution of radioactive cannabinoids in the plasma was similar in the two groups. The authors concluded that frequent use of marijuana does not alter the response quantitatively or qualitatively to intravenous THC-Δ-9; i.e., neither tolerance nor sensitivity to the THC-Δ-9 developed.

Renault et al. (159) administered small doses of marijuana to young adults for a 10-day period preceded and followed by 3 days of placebo. Four subjects received the equivalent of 6.5 mg THC-Δ-9 twice a day and four received the equivalent of 12.25 mg THC-Δ-9 twice a day each day. Time estimation was disrupted in subjects receiving the higher dose but gradually improved during the smoking period. Two of the three subjects receiving the higher doses (12.25 mg THC-Δ-9) did not tolerate it well, which led to a change in the experimental procedure.

In all these studies—except that of Williams et al. (205)—subjects were either infrequent users or short-term heavy users. By definition, tolerance is related to frequency and duration of use. In the present study the Greek subjects had used hashish at least twice daily for an average of 23 years. In this report we examine the effect of abrupt cessation of use for a brief period and the effect of reintroduction of use on some aspects of mental functioning.

REVIEW OF PROCEDURES

Sixteen subjects smoked placebo for 3 days and marijuana for 3 days. All smoking was *ad libitum*. Half of the subjects received placebo first and then marijuana (order 1); the other half received marijuana then placebo (order 2). On each day there were two smoking periods 4.5 hr apart.

Subjects were inpatients for the 6-day period. Marijuana contained 2.6% THC-Δ-9. Cigarettes were 1 g each, containing 26 mg THC-Δ-9. Two days prior to the testing period, all subjects smoked marijuana *ad libitum* as outpatients to ensure at least a minimum consumption of marijuana.

Tests of mental functioning were administered 2 hr 10 min after the first smoking on each day. The testing period was 30 min. On the third and sixth days the same tests were administered immediately after the second smoking.

Test Battery

Three of the tests had been used previously during the acute phase and are discussed in Chapter 11 (48). These were:

1. *Serial sevens:* The subject is given a number between 99 and 104 and is required to subtract seven from that number to the point that further subtraction is not possible. The time to complete the task and number of errors are combined to yield a fault index.

2. *Barrage de signe:* (a) This is an alertness test somewhat similar to the digit symbol substitute task (DSST). Subjects are given a sheet with rows of symbols. Three symbols at the top of the page serve as standards. Subjects are required to cross out as rapidly as possible the symbols on the sheet which are the same as the three standards. There is a 1.5-min limit on this task. The score is the number correct minus 0.5 point for each error. (b) In addition to being administered as above, the task was presented a second time with a simultaneous addition task to make it more difficult. The second presentation required the subject to cross out as above (step a) and at the same time to add three to a number starting between 20 and 30.

3. *Time estimation:* The subject was asked to estimate the duration of the 5-min number ordination task (described below).

The new tests included:

4. *DSST:* This is a subtest of the WAIS and administered in the same way as in the WAIS. The subject is presented with a sheet on which are the digits 1 through 9. Each digit has a corresponding symbol below it. The subject is then presented with rows of digits and is required to fill in the symbol associated with each digit with the original digit-symbol pairs in view. The score is the number of correct associations completed within a 90-sec period.

5. *Number ordination:* The subject is presented with lists of seven digits in random order and must write them in increasing order as quickly as possible. The score is the total number of digits correctly ordered during a 5-min period.

For the 2.5-hr postsmoking testing period, data were analyzed in separate three-way analyses of variance with order (placebo-marijuana, marijuana-placebo), drug (placebo, marijuana), and days (1, 2, 3) as the main variables. For the immediate postsmoking testing period, data were analyzed in two-way analyses of variance, with order and drug as the main variables.

RESULTS

The reader is referred to Chapter 16 for discussion of the smoking data for this phase.

Two hours postsmoking

For comparison with the psychological test performance data, the number of cigarettes smoked during the first smoking session as a function of the order of drug administration is shown in Fig. 17-1 (Left).

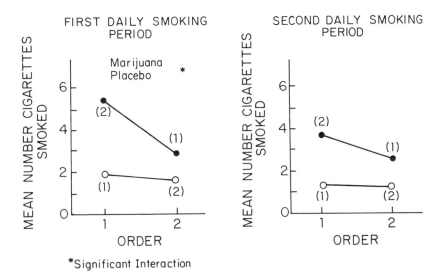

*Significant Interaction

FIG. 17-1. Left: Mean number of marijuana and placebo cigarettes consumed in each order during the first daily smoking period. Data is summed over days. **Right:** Mean number of marijuana and placebo cigarettes consumed in each order on days 3 and 6 during the second daily smoking period. In both figures (1) indicates the substance administered during the first 3-day period in each order; (2) indicates the substance administered during the second 3-day period. The asterisk (*) indicates that the interaction between order of drug administration and drug is significant.

Serial Sevens

In the serial sevens test there is a significant interaction between drugs and the order in which they are administered. Performance is impaired after smoking marijuana when marijuana administration precedes placebo administration. However, when marijuana conditions follow placebo administration, performance is slightly better than it is in the placebo conditions (Fig. 17-2, left). This interaction indicates a practice effect. Performance is better during the second 3-day period regardless of the drug administered. If subjects smoked placebo first and then marijuana, performance is better in the marijuana condition (subjects smoked an average of 140 mg THC-Δ-9); if subjects smoked marijuana and then placebo, performance is better in the placebo conditions. The practice effect is considerably greater in the latter condition, i.e., marijuana to placebo.

Barrage de Signe

(a) There is a significant interaction between drugs and their order of administration in the *barrage de signe* test which suggests a large practice effect. Performance is better in the marijuana condition when it follows placebo and worse when it precedes placebo (Fig. 17-3A). The

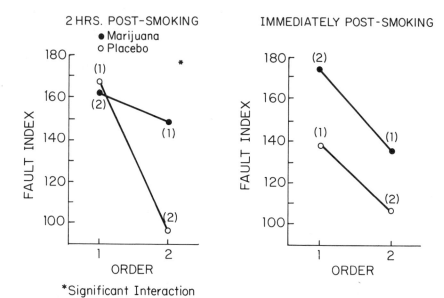

*Significant Interaction

FIG. 17-2. Left: Serial sevens. Mean error score 2 hr after the first daily smoking session (summed over days) as a function of the order of drug administration. **Right:** Mean error score measured on days 3 and 6 immediately after the second daily smoking period as a function of the order of drug administration. In both figures (1) indicates the substance administered during the first 3-day period in each order; (2) indicates the substance administered during the second 3-day period. The asterisk (*) indicates that the interaction between order of drug administration and drug is significant.

practice effect is so predominant that during the marijuana smoking days which follow placebo subjects smoke an average of 140 mg THC-Δ-9 but their performance is considerably better than it is on the marijuana days which precede placebo, when subjects smoked an average of 75 mg THC-Δ-9.

(b) When the addition task is added to *barrage de signe*, the same pattern of results are obtained as when *barrage de signe* is presented alone, but the magnitude of response is lower (Fig. 17-3B).

Time Estimation

There are no significant effects in the task of estimating a 5-min period (Fig. 17-4, left). There is a tendency to slight overestimation in all conditions (i.e., estimates are greater than 5 min); this tendency remains stable over days in the marijuana conditions even though there are significantly fewer cigarettes smoked over these days.

DSST

There is a significant interaction between drugs and their order of adminis-tration in the DSST, as was the case in the serial sevens and *barrage de*

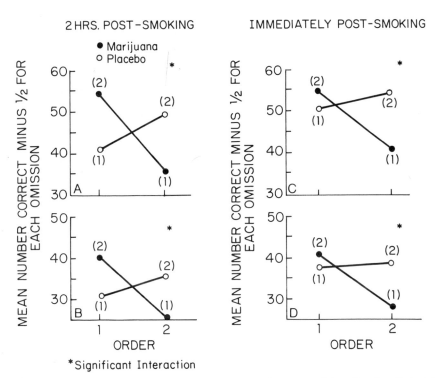

FIG. 17-3. *Barrage de Signe.* **A:** Mean correct performance 2 hr after the first daily smoking period (summed over days) as a function of the order of drug administration. **B:** Mean correct performance in the *Barrage de Signe* task measured while subjects were engaged in a simultaneous addition task. This was recorded 2 hr after the first daily smoking period (summed over days). **C:** Mean correct performance on days 3 and 6 measured immediately after the second daily smoking period as a function of order of drug administration. **D:** Mean correct performance on days 3 and 6 in the *Barrage de Signe* task measured while subjects were engaged in a simultaneous addition task. This measurement occurred immediately after the second smoking period. (1) indicates the substance administered during the first 3-day period in each order; (2) indicates the substance administered during the second 3-day period. The asterisk (*) indicates that the interaction between order of drug administration and drug is significant.

signe tasks. There is a large practice effect; performance always improves during the second 3-day smoking period, regardless of the drug administered. Performance is better in the marijuana condition when it follows placebo, and impaired when it precedes placebo (Fig. 17-5, left). Even though there is considerably more marijuana smoked after the placebo period than before it, performance after the placebo period is considerably better than it is before the placebo period.

Number Ordination

In regard to number ordination there is again a significant interaction between drugs and their order of presentation. There is a large practice

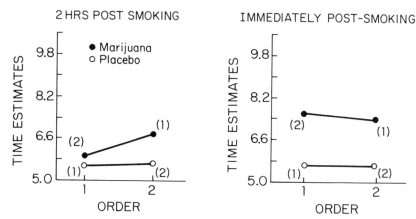

FIG. 17-4. Time estimation. **Left:** Mean time estimates of a 5-min task measured 2 hr after the first daily smoking period (summed over days) as a function of the order of drug administration. **Right:** Mean time estimates of a 5-min task measured immediately after the second smoking period on days 3 and 6 as a function of the order of drug administration.

(1): The substance administered during the first 3-day period in each order; (2): the substance administered during the second 3-day period.

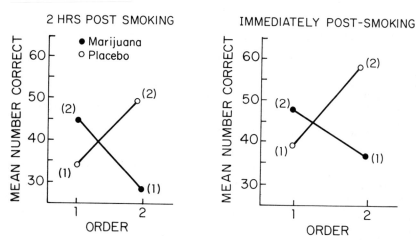

FIG. 17-5. DSST. **Left:** Mean number of symbols correctly associated with digits measured 2 hr after the first daily smoking period as a function of the order of drug administration (data are summed over days). **Right:** Mean number of symbols correctly associated with digits measured immediately after the second smoking period on days 3 and 6.

(1) Indicates the substance administered during the first 3-day period in each order; (2) indicates the substance administered during the second 3-day period.

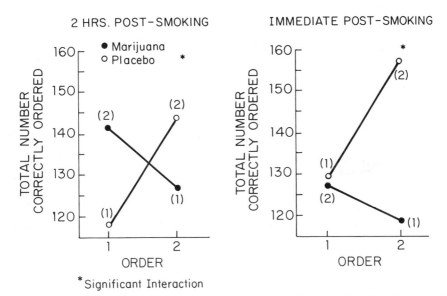

FIG. 17-6. Number ordination. **Left:** Mean number of digits correctly ordered measured 2 hr after the first daily smoking session as a function of the order of administration of drugs. **Right:** Mean number of digits correctly ordered measured immediately after the second smoking period on days 3 and 6. In both figures (1) indicates the substance administered during the first 3-day period in each order; (2) indicates the substance administered during the second 3-day period. The asterisk (*) indicates that the interaction between order of drug administration and drug is significant.

effect which is so predominant that performance during marijuana smoking days—when the marijuana period follows placebo (Fig. 17-6, left) is as good as it is during placebo smoking days.

Summary

In serial sevens, *barrage de signe,* DSST, and number ordination, there is a significant interaction between drugs and their order of presentation. In all instances the interaction indicates the presence of a practice effect, which 2 hr after smoking is predominant over the drug effect.

Immediate Postsmoking Period

For comparison with the psychological test data, the number of cigarettes smoked during the second smoking period on days 3 and 6 as a function of order of drug administration is shown in Fig. 17-1 (right).

Serial Sevens

Performance of serial sevens is significantly impaired after marijuana administration (Fig. 17-2, right).

Barrage de Signe

(a) There is a significant interaction between drugs and their order of administration in regard to *barrage de signe*. When marijuana administration follows placebo administration, performance is slightly improved in the marijuana conditions compared to placebo conditions (Fig. 17-3C), but when marijuana precedes placebo performance is impaired.

(b) When the addition task is presented with *barrage de signe,* the same results are obtained as when *barrage de signe* is presented alone; i.e., there is a significant interaction between drugs and their order of administration (Fig. 17-3D).

Time Estimation

There are no significant effects in the time estimation (5 min) task. There is a tendency for time to be overestimated after marijuana, but the difference between marijuana and placebo conditions is not significant (Fig. 17-4, right).

DSST

In the DSST there is a significant interaction between drugs and their order of administration, as was the case with *barrage de signe*. Performance after marijuana administration is better than after placebo administration when marijuana follows placebo, and impaired when marijuana precedes placebo (Fig. 17-5, right).

Number Ordination

The interaction between drugs and their order of administration is significant in the number ordination task. Performance after placebo administration is better when it follows marijuana administration. When placebo precedes marijuana, performance is the same for both drugs. (Fig. 17-6, right).

Summary

Performance in all tasks except time estimation is always better after the administration of placebo than after marijuana smoking. This is reflected in a significant drug effect in all tasks. However, the interaction between drug and the order of its administration also indicates large practice effects which are less predominant than the drug effect.

Comparisons Between Immediate and Two-Hour Postsmoking Performances

The comparisons between postsmoking performances are shown in Figs. 17-2 through 17-6. In these figures the immediate postsmoking data are based on performance on the third and sixth days of each order. The 2-hr postsmoking data are based on a summary over 3 days for each drug in each order, i.e., days 1–3 placebo and days 4–6 marijuana; days 1–3 marijuana and days 4–6 placebo. Task performance 2 hr after the first smoking and immediately after the second smoking are similar in magnitude. To ensure that these data are not misleading, mean performances on the third and sixth days 2 hr postsmoking were calculated. They are similar and sometimes identical to the average over days.

DISCUSSION

Psychological test performance after smoking 140 mg THC-Δ-9 is either better or similar to performance after smoking placebo depending on the sequence of drug administration. This equivalence occurs both immediately and 2 hr after smoking. The difference in the two testing periods is that immediately after smoking there is a tendency for the drug effect to limit the practice effect, whereas 2 hr after smoking the practice effect is predominant. The major exception to improved performance after previous practice is in serial sevens, where there is an increase in error scores after marijuana administration when tested immediately after smoking.

In *barrage de signe*, DSST, and number ordination, the significant interaction between drugs and their order of administration indicates that the practice effect is evident after the administration of marijuana. Subjects who smoke marijuana after placebo even though they smoke one-third more than those who smoke marijuana before placebo perform better than the latter, indicating that they are benefiting from their previous experience under placebo. Performance after placebo also improves when subjects have practiced previously on marijuana. The improvement from marijuana to placebo is always greater than from placebo to marijuana, however, indicating that cannabis does inhibit test performance.

In some instances performance after smoking marijuana is the same in the placebo-marijuana order as after placebo, suggesting the possibility that marijuana does not affect performance. When interpreted with the data of the marijuana-placebo order, however, it is probable that the practice effect in the placebo-marijuana order cannot be exhibited fully because of the direct effect of cannabis. Thus in contrast to the data of the 2-hr postsmoking testing period, the practice effect immediately after smoking is overshadowed by the drug effect.

These data are in contrast to reports of state-dependent learning (137–139,176). This theory claims that after learning a task in a particular state performance of that task can best be reproduced when the subject is in that state again. Thus recall of learning which takes place under the influence of a drug is impaired when it is reproduced in a nondrug state. Stillman et al. (176) reported state-dependent effects after the administration of social doses of marijuana (7.5 mg THC-Δ-9).

Although the design necessary to test state-dependent effects was not used in this study (i.e., marijuana-marijuana, placebo-marijuana, marijuana-placebo, placebo-placebo), it is clear that in most tests there was obvious and significant improvement from nondrug to drug state (placebo-marijuana: order 1) and from drug to nondrug state (marijuana-placebo: order 2), which is typically not obtained in state-dependent studies in which the subject is impaired when he performs in a state different from the one in which he learned. The differences in performances observed in these Greek subjects and those observed, for example, by Stillman et al. (176) may be due to differences in populations and experience with the drug. Stillman's subjects were young adult volunteers who had smoked marijuana a minimum of six times.

In the American culture most users smoke marijuana to get "high." In the Greek subjects, hashish is part of the life style and may serve a more adaptive function. In Chapter 6 we related the reasons given for continued use of hashish by Greek subjects. They describe relaxation, working better, and increased problem-solving ability after smoking hashish. In other cultures there is a different set of expectations associated with cannabis use and different drug effects (18,166). Jamaicans, for example, use ganja to increase concentration, increase work output, and to impart a sense of well-being. American users report an awareness of the cognitive and performance deficits produced by marijuana and consequent interference with their work (165). Jamaicans take ganja to enhance work, but the work of ganja users is not intellectual but manual labor, which cannabis may make more tolerable. This use of cannabis to make tedious work more tolerable is true for the Greek sample also. Nevertheless, these men perform very well in the tests of mental functioning considering the large quantities of THC-Δ-9 they consume. It is probable that their performance reflects their long years of use and adaptation to the effects of cannabis (200). There is a tolerance evidenced by these subjects which does not exhibit withdrawal effects (e.g., in terms of disturbing concentration) on these tests. Subjects consuming the equivalent of 140 mg THC-Δ-9 after a 3-day abstinence period (Order 1) perform as well, and even better, than subjects consuming less and not exposed to the 3-day abstinence period (Order 2).

SUMMARY

Sixteen subjects smoked marijuana *ad libitum* twice a day for a 3-day period. A 3-day *ad libitum* placebo smoking condition either preceded or followed the marijuana conditions. The psychological test battery was administered after both smokings: 2 hr after the first smoking on each day, and immediately after the second smoking on days 3 and 6.

After the first smoking there was a drug effect on serial sevens, *barrage de signe*, DSST, and number ordination tasks. There was no effect on time estimation. The drug effect, however, was related to the order of administration of marijuana relative to placebo; i.e., when marijuana was administered after placebo, task performance on marijuana smoking days was better than on placebo smoking days, and task performance was worse on marijuana smoking days when marijuana preceded placebo.

The level of marijuana task performance when it followed placebo was better than the level of performance achieved when it preceded placebo. A similar effect was observed on placebo smoking days when placebo followed marijuana; task performance was better than when the placebo condition preceded marijuana.

When the test battery was administered immediately after smoking, there was a drug effect on the *barrage de signe*, DSST, and number ordination tasks similar to that observed 2 hr after smoking; i.e., the effects were related to the order of administration of marijuana. Performance on these three tasks was as good or better on the marijuana smoking days than on the placebo smoking days when the marijuana condition followed the placebo condition and impaired when it preceded placebo. In the serial sevens task, performance was impaired after smoking marijuana regardless of the order of marijuana administration. There was no effect on time estimation.

The relationship between marijuana effect and its order of administration relative to placebo suggests the existence of practice effects (positive transfer), which are observed both immediately as well as 2 hr after smoking. The positive transfer from placebo to marijuana 2 hr after smoking is greater than it is immediately after smoking, indicating a less intense but still-present drug effect 2 hr after smoking. This is consistent with the time course of the marijuana effect.

18
Withdrawal from Cannabis: Psychophysiological Changes

John Boulougouris, Aris Liakos, Costas Stefanis,
Rhea Dornbush, and C. P. Panayiotopoulos

Psychophysiological and mood effects have been extensively studied after a single administration of marijuana, as well as after daily administration for periods varying from 10 to 52 days. These studies employ either irregular or frequent users who have as-yet short-term experience with the drug (50,51,82,89,93,126,127,142,160,162,163,193,194). The most consistent finding is a significant and dose-related increase in heart rate (51,193) and a feeling of being "high" (126,127,200). With daily administration for at least 21 days, the heart rate increases after smoking during the first 1–2 weeks. Thereafter the amount of increase diminishes until the heart rate does not differ from presmoking levels (50,111,126,127,205), although Renault et al. (159) found heart rate increases during each of 10 days of smoking. It is difficult to judge whether these changes in heart rate represent tolerance, habituation, or fatigue in the experimental situation, as no study used adequate placebo control groups.

Smokers in North America are said to seek the feeling of the "high" when they use marijuana. The "high" is a widely used but poorly understood term. Drug users are vague in their description of the state, although the existence of the "high" based on self-ratings from simply constructed scales has been documented during acute use (126,127,194). In one experiment separate ratings were obtained for "high," the "pleasantness" of the high, and the heart rate. The "high" increased linearly with heart rate. Pleasantness, however, increased with heart rate only until approximately 100 beats/min. Thereafter it decreased with increasing heart rate. It is possible that heart rate is used as the cue to regulate the dosage under the usual smoking conditions. With daily smoking of a standard dose under laboratory conditions, the subjective effects usually decrease—a response that may be related more to the experimental conditions (confinement) than to tolerance (49). In an *ad libitum* study for 21 days, Mendelson et al. (126,127) reported a tendency for heavy users to rate themselves less "high" as they continued to smoke, even as they increased their daily marijuana intake. In these smokers heart rate decreased during the experiment when it was recorded 25 min after smoking.

EEG effects have also been well defined in acute use. In short-term users

(116,194) and long-term users (Chapter 12), particularly when using the refined techniques of computer analysis, there is an increase in the amount of alpha activity; a decrease in average frequency and in beta activity; an increase in latencies in various components of the visual, auditory, and somatic sensory evoked responses; and an increased amplitude of the contingent negative variation.

The effects of marijuana on other physiological measures has not been as well studied. Pupil size, respiration rate, body temperature, and blood pressure are unchanged by cannabis, although blood pressure may be lowered with high doses (81,85,116). Peripheral vasodilation, patchy flushing of the face, and facial pallor have been noted in hashish users (4,86). Peripheral blood flow increases when measured by plethysmography (10).

The literature related to physiological dependence on marijuana in longterm users is limited. To study the withdrawal symptoms after cessation of marijuana smoking, various psychophysiological parameters were measured during a 3-day abstinence period and were compared to a 3-day period of marijuana use.

REVIEW OF PROCEDURES

During this study (described in Chapter 4) the subjects smoked marijuana and placebo on an *ad libitum* basis. The amounts of the prepared cigarettes smoked were recorded. The physiological and subjective measurements taken 4 hr after the first smoking each day and immediately after the second smoking on days 2 and 5 were similar to those recorded in the acute inhalation studies: pulse rate, finger pulse volume, respiration rate, temperature, blood pressure, and *mastura* (''high'') self-ratings. Just before the second smoking on days 2 and 5, and also five minutes after that smoking session, the pupil size was measured. The recording of these measures lasted 30 min, and the techniques are described in Chapter 15.

Data Processing

Three-way analyses of variance were performed for the data obtained 4 hr postsmoking. Order (placebo-marijuana, marijuana-placebo), drug (placebo, marijuana), and days (1, 2, 3) were the main variables. Three-way analyses of variance were performed for the data obtained immediately postsmoking on the second and fifth day. Order, drug, and time were the main variables. As the recording was for 30 min, six 5-min averages were obtained.

Analyses of the quantities of cigarettes smoked during each smoking period are described in Chapter 16. To evaluate physiological data, smoking data are presented where appropriate.

RESULTS

Four Hours Postsmoking

Heart Rate

Four hours after smoking marijuana, the pulse rate had not yet returned to baseline and was higher than the placebo values. There was an interaction between drug (marijuana and placebo) and the days of smoking: Pulse rate remained at baseline levels on the 3 days when placebo was smoked but decreased progressively on the 3 days marijuana was smoked (Fig. 18-1, left). The number of cigarettes consumed increased slightly from day 1 to day 2 and then decreased to its lowest amount on day 3 (Fig. 18-1, right).

EEG Data

Although there are some differences in the abundance of some EEG frequencies after smoking marijuana, there were no effects related to the sequence or the days of smoking. There was a greater amount of 7.5–10.5 Hz and a lesser amount of 15.5–24.5 Hz after smoking marijuana compared to the amounts elicited after smoking placebo. These changes are similar to those seen in the acute smoking experiences in these subjects (Chapter 12).

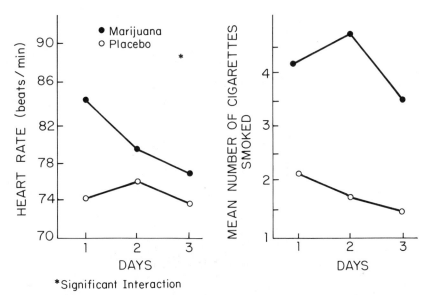

FIG. 18-1. Heart-rate. **Left:** Mean heart-rate displayed over days. Data were obtained 4 hr after the first daily smoking session. **Right:** Mean number of cigarettes smoked during the first daily smoking session displayed over days. The asterisk (*) indicates that the interaction between order of drug administration and drug itself is significant.

TABLE 18-1. *Withdrawal phase (N = 12): visual evoked responses*

| | Latency (msec) | | | | Amplitude (μV) | | | |
| | Placebo | | Drug | | Placebo | | Drug | |
Component	Pre	Post	Pre	Post	Pre	Post	Pre	Post
P_1	71.5 ± 16.8	73.3 ± 17.0	70.4 ± 23.2	70.5 ± 17.4	8.7 ± 6.4	7.6 ± 5.4	9.4 ± 6.6	8.3 ± 6.1
N_2	90.8 ± 20.6	93.5 ± 21.5	93.0 ± 21.1	94.3 ± 19.9	12.9 ± 9.25	11.2 ± 7.0	13.9 ± 10.0	11.4 ± 7.1
P_2	114.3 ± 16.8	117.4 ± 18.7	120.0 ± 17.1	122.5 ± 16.9	18.8 ± 10.1	17.4 ± 8.1	21.1 ± 11.6	17.9 ± 9.4
N_3	162.1 ± 16.2	163.8 ± 17.4	166.5 ± 20.1	167.3 ± 19.1	26.2 ± 10.4	24.8 ± 10.8	25.1 ± 9.9	23.8 ± 9.8

Results are given as the mean ± SD.

Respiration Rate

There was an increase in respiration rate during the second 3-day period in both the placebo-marijuana and marijuana-placebo orders (Fig. 18-2, left), and no change was drug-related. For comparison purposes, the mean number of cigarettes smoked is shown in Fig. 18-2 (Right).

Temperature: There is a significant drug and sequence by drug interaction. Temperature is higher after marijuana administration. In the interaction temperature is higher for marijuana conditions in both order 1 and order 2 compared to placebo conditions in each sequence. It is highest for the marijuana condition when marijuana occupies the second 3-day period. As considerably more marijuana was smoked in order 1 than in order 2 this suggests that temperature fluctuations may be directly influenced by quantities of THC-Δ-9 consumed.

Finger pulse volume: There are significant drug, sequence by drug, and sequence by drug by day interactions. Width measurements are lower after smoking marijuana in order 1. In order 2 marijuana and placebo measurements are similar. In the triple interaction, the pattern of response over days for placebo when it occupies the first 3-day period (order 1) is similar to the pattern of response for marijuana when it occupies the first 3-day period (order 2); and likewise there are similar patterns for both drug conditions over days when each occupies the second 3-day testing period.

Pupil size: No differences between marijuana smoking and placebo were observed.

Mastura

Mastura measurements were recorded immediately after smoking on all days. Measurements were recorded after both the first and second smoking periods on each day. Since placebo was rated zero, these ratings were not included in this analysis. The three main variables are order (placebo-marijuana, marijuana-placebo), days (1, 2, 3), and smoking (first, second).

Mastura ratings after smoking marijuana following an abstinence period were higher (5.0) than when smoking before abstinence (2.7). More marijuana was smoked during the period which followed abstinence (4.6 versus 2.7 cigarettes). Ratings were higher after the second smoking session (4.1) than after the first (3.6), although less marijuana was smoked during the second session (3.1 cigarettes) than during the first (4.1 cigarettes). This suggests that the quantities consumed during the first and second sessions may be additive.

The subjects correctly assessed the placebo cigarette and valued it little. When the 3-day marijuana period followed the abstinence period, however, *mastura* ratings were higher than when the marijuana period preceded abstinence (Fig. 18-3). This difference is related to the quantity of THC-Δ-9 consumed (Fig. 18-2, right). A greater number of marijuana cigarettes were smoked during the period that followed abstinence than during that which preceded abstinence.

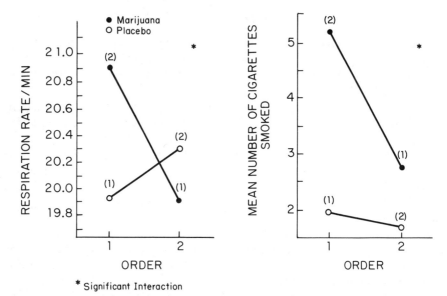

* Significant Interaction

FIG. 18-2. Respiration rate. **Left:** Mean respiration rate displayed over days. Data were obtained 4 hr after the first daily smoking session. **Right:** Mean number cigarettes smoked during first daily smoking session as a function of order of drug administration. (Data are summed over days). In both figures (1) indicates the substance administered first in each order; (2) indicates the substance administered second in each order. The asterisk(*) indicates that the interaction between order of drug administration and drug itself is significant.

FIG. 18-3. *Mastura ratings.* Mean *mastura* (mood) values as a function of order of drug administration. (Data are summed over days)

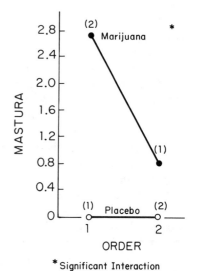

* Significant Interaction

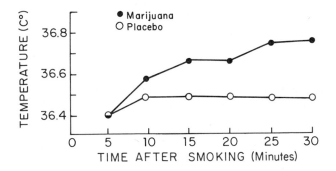

FIG. 18-4. Temperature. Mean temperature (°C) measured for the 30 min immediately after the smoking session.

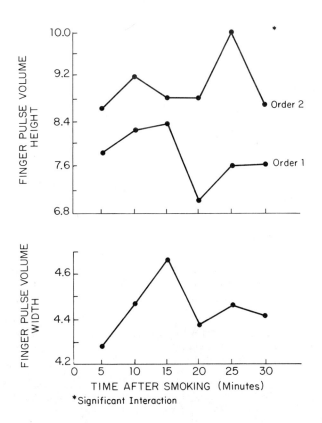

FIG. 18-5. Finger pulse volume (FPV). **Top:** Height measurements recorded for a 30-min period immediately after the second daily smoking session on days 2 and 5. **Right:** Width measurements recorded for a 30-min period immediately after the second daily smoking session on days 2 and 5. The asterisk (*) indicates a significant order by time interaction.

Blood Pressure

Both systolic and diastolic pressures rise on day 2 and fall on day 3 when smoking marijuana. With placebo, blood pressure measurements decrease consecutively over days. (Fig. 18-6, left and right). The number of marijuana cigarettes smoked increases on day 2 suggesting that blood pressure (as temperature) may fluctuate in relation to the quantity of THC-Δ-9 smoked.

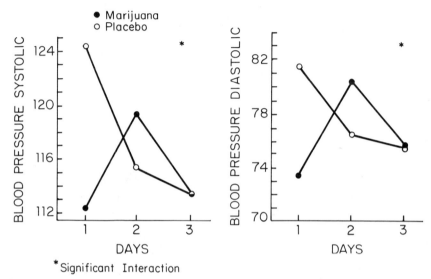

*Significant Interaction

FIG. 18-6. Blood pressure. **Left:** Systolic blood pressure recorded immediately after smoking on days 2 and 5. Data are displayed over days. **Right:** Diastolic blood pressure recorded immediately after smoking on days 2 and 5. Data are displayed over days. The asterisk (*) indicates that the drug by day interaction is significant.

Drachmas

Subjects were asked to indicate how much they would pay (in drachmas) for what they smoked. The assessments were made immediately after each smoking. As placebo values were effectively zero, these were not included in the analyses. In a three-way analysis of variance, the main variables (order, day, and smoking period) each showed an effect. The values were higher when the marijuana smoking period followed the abstinence period (26.6 drachmas) than when marijuana smoking preceded abstinence (14.0). Indeed, more marijuana was smoked when the smoking period followed abstinence than when it preceded it. Values decreased consistently during the 3-day smoking period (24.1, 19.4, and 17.5 drachmas, respectively) as did the quantity of marijuana consumed (3.7, 3.8, 3.4 cigarettes, respectively). In contrast to *mastura,* drachma values were higher after the first smoking session than after the second (22.1 and 18.5, respectively); more marijuana was smoked during the first session than during the second (4.1 and 3.1 cigarettes, respectively).

Immediate Postsmoking Measurements

Heart Rate

The pulse rate is higher after marijuana administration and decreases during the 30-min recording period. Although the number of cigarettes consumed is greater during the 3-day period following abstinence than the 3-day period preceding abstinence, the pulse rate does not reflect this difference (Fig. 18-7, left and right).

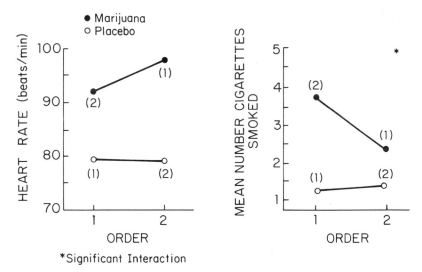

*Significant Interaction

FIG. 18-7. Heart-rate. **Left:** Mean heart-rate response measured immediately after smoking on days 2 and 5 as a function of order of drug administration. **Right:** Mean number of cigarettes smoked during the second daily smoking session on days 2 and 5 as a function of order of drug administration.

Respiration Rate

There are no effects on the respiration rate.

Temperature

For placebo conditions the temperature increases after the first 5-min evaluation and remains stable during the remaining measurement period (to 30 min). For marijuana conditions the temperature increases consistently during the 30-min measurement (Fig. 18-4).

Finger Pulse Volume

Separate analyses were done for height and width measurements. There are uneven and inconsistent changes in both measures (Fig. 18-5, left). All height measurements in order 2 are higher than those in order 1. The tendency in order 2 is to increase, and in order 2 to decrease. For the width measurements the time variable is significant (Fig. 18-5, right).

Comparisons Between Immediate Postsmoking and Four-Hour Postsmoking Measurements

As the variables in each recording period were not always the same and the same interactions were not significant, it is difficult to evaluate the differences in measurements. No statistical analyses were performed on these comparisons.

An analysis was performed on the *mastura* recordings comparing ratings immediately postsmoking with those obtained 4 hr postsmoking. Both ratings were made after the first smoking period. This was the only variable for which such measurements were obtained. The analysis was a three-way analysis of variance; order, day, and time (immediate, 4 hr) are the main variables. *Mastura* ratings are higher after marijuana administration when it follows placebo than they are when marijuana precedes placebo. In addition, ratings are higher immediately after smoking than they are 4 hr after smoking.

Placebo measurements show either no increment or minimum fluctuation in pulse rate, temperature, and *mastura* ratings. There is a consistent decrease in blood pressure values, suggesting an habituation effect. There is also a consistent increment in respiration rate, suggesting that the increment observed after marijuana may not be a drug effect only but that it may be related to some aspect of the experimental situation such as annoyance, fatigue, habituation, etc.

DISCUSSION

These observations reveal some differences in blood pressure, heart rate, and temperature, for example, which may be related to an abstinence phenomenon. If tolerance development is a feature of long-term cannabis use, it develops slowly, showing the characteristics of tolerance similar to those of alcohol and tobacco. In these dependencies, withdrawal symptoms are expressed slowly and without the dramatic quality expressed for the withdrawal to opioids, barbiturates, and amphetamine. In the present study of long-term cannabis users, the withdrawal period was 3 days. During the first day of smoking marijuana, the subjects smoked more cigarettes than later, and some of the physiological measures reflected a greater effect. At best, these findings are suggestive of a withdrawal syndrome. The failure to demonstrate it more clearly may be a reflection of the degree of tolerance and dependence development, as well as the short period of observation in this study.

Jones (92) reported the appearance of physical dependence with a withdrawal syndrome similar to that produced by CNS general depressants after the cessation of a 10- to 18-day period of THC-Δ-9 administration. Jones administered a total of 210 mg THC-Δ-9 orally during each 24-hr period, with 30 mg administered every 4 hr. This finding of dependence was observed after the continuous and consistent dosing of THC-Δ-9 in a fashion similar to a medication schedule or an animal bar-pressing paradigm, rather than patterns of social use. Cannabis users (Greek or American) do not usually follow such a rigid and frequent schedule. Others have also had difficulty in defining a withdrawal syndrome in studies of either single administration in regular users or daily administration for longer periods (10,84,85,200,201).

19

Withdrawal from Cannabis: Laboratory Tests and Clinical Observations

Costas Ballas, John Boulougouris, Aris Liakos, and Costas Stefanis

The existence of a cannabis abstinence syndrome is ill-defined. Jones and Benowitz (93) reported physical withdrawal symptoms after the administration of high doses of cannabis, and these observations are similar to those of others (14,205). The findings are less intense than those seen after opiate withdrawal (142). Frazer (61a) described several cases of acute psychosis associated with the withdrawal of cannabis indica from addicts, which he observed during a military campaign in the Far East. The cases appeared in the first four days, principally in Indian troops. The presenting symptom was irritability, culminating in outbursts of violence. Under medical supervision the men became quiet and rational, and seemed mildly depressed. But 48 to 72 hours after their return to their units, the men had other outbursts of impulsivity, and some had acute psychotic episodes lasting 3 to 6 weeks. Bensusen (14) reported that seven ganja smokers developed anxiety, restlessness, sweating, hypotension, and muscular aches after withdrawal of cannabis.

Mild irritability is the only symptom of withdrawal from the sustained use of cannabis, according to McGlothlin and West (122), who reject the notion of physical dependence and suggest only that psychological dependence may occur. Grinspoon (68) states "There is now an abundance of evidence that marijuana is not an addictive drug. Cessation of its use produces no withdrawal symptoms, nor does a user feel any need to increase the dosage as he becomes accustomed to the drug." Williams et al. (205) reported restlessness, insomnia, anorexia and increased perspiration to occur on the second day after the abrupt withdrawal of pyrahexyl, a synthetic cannabis-like substance. Others have reported similar symptoms in marijuana users, with the symptoms being relieved by alcohol or barbiturates (91).

In animal studies, monkeys have been given 0.1 to 0.4 mg per kg doses of THC-Δ-9 daily for a month and then developed yawning, anorexia, pilo-erection, irritability, photophobia and tremors on withdrawal (96).

In this chapter, we present the observations in the medical, laboratory, and behavioral observations during the acute withdrawal study in long-term hashish users.

147

METHODS

Neurological and Laboratory Tests: A brief neurological examination was done every day, three and a half hours after the first smoking of cigarettes. Reflexes (corneal and deep tendon), vibration sense, coordination tests, and eye movements for nystagmus were examined. Muscle strength was measured with a hand dynamometer and tremor was measured with a tremorgraph.

A chest x-ray and blood samples were taken on the third day of each three-day sequence, two hours after smoking. The blood was examined for liver function tests, blood counts, sedimentation rate, blood sugar, uric acid, lactic acid, cholesterol, non-esterified lipid acids, 17-ketosteroids, and catecholamines (epinephrine and norepinephrine).

Rating scales: Symptom self rating scales (10-point) were used each day, two hours after the first smoking of the day. Subjects rated anxiety, depression, fatigue, restlessness, irritability, and sexual desire. Also rated, but on a three-point scale, were the presence of constipation, flatulence, abdominal pain, and the degree of appetite.

Psychiatric Interview: A structured psychiatric interview was conducted four hours after smoking on the first and third days of each three day sequence. The following were assessed: general behavior, body image, imagination, perceptual distortions, bodily sensations, hallucinations, the quality, quantity and rate of speech, and the degree of suspiciousness.

Twice a day each subject was interviewed by a psychiatrist and a social worker who evaluated the subject's adjustment on the ward, their motility, cooperation with the staff, talkativeness, and the presence of any 'abnormal' behavior such as irritability or outbursts of aggressivity.

RESULTS

The subjects were relaxed, talkative, and willing to participate on the day of admission. During the experimental periods, the symptom ratings showed no differences in irritability, depression, anxiety, or restlessness. The ratings for all symptoms including fatigue are generally low for both withdrawal and active drug periods, being at or below 2 units on the 10-point scale. Fatigue ratings were highest on the first day of the smoking period and decreased on days 2 and 3. The ratings were lowest on day 1 of the withdrawal period and increased on days 2 and 3.

Small differences were also noted between smoking and withdrawal periods in the ratings of constipation, flatulence, appetite and cramps, these symptoms being greater during withdrawal.

In total psychopathology score, measured each day during smoking and post-smoking periods, there is a tendency towards more abnormal psychopathology during marijuana smoking during the first day than during the last when measured immediately (15 min) after smoking; and the opposite trend when measured four hours after smoking.

In adjustment on the ward, the subjects were better adjusted while they smoked marijuana irrespective of the order of smoking. Those subjects who started with the sequence of placebo followed by marijuana became hostile when they realized that they were not smoking marijuana, and became more cooperative when marijuana was smoked.

Subjects who started with the sequence of smoking marijuana first followed by placebo, had a more positive attitude throughout the experiment. The staff assessed patient cooperation as better when users were smoking marijuana than when they were smoking placebo. Eleven of 16 users were more talkative when smoking marijuana than placebo, and almost all subjects showed increased motor activity with marijuana. Irritability was greater with placebo. Neither aggressive behavior nor outbursts of violence were seen. Two of the subjects exhibited abnormal behavior while smoking marijuana. One was demanding, restless, and paranoid; the other described visual and auditory hallucinations, but claimed these symptoms were not disturbing. Both continued the experiments and did not require any medication on the ward.

Throughout the study periods, the laboratory and neurological examinations remained within the normal baseline limits.

SUMMARY

No overt clinical symptoms or laboratory findings indicating a cannabis physical withdrawal syndrome were seen in this study. Our results are consistent with the findings of others (36,127).

20

Study of Long-Term Hashish Users in Greece: Summary and Discussion

Max Fink

These studies were undertaken in Greece to determine if the long-term use of hashish is associated with behavioral, medical, neurological, psychological, or social deficits; if tolerance, dependence, or a withdrawal syndrome were demonstrable; and to define the pharmacological-behavioral relations resulting from hashish, marijuana, and pure THC-Δ-9 consumption. The studies were designed in 1970, and the questions posed reflect the concerns of cannabis researchers at that time:

Is prolonged cannabis use associated with brain damage, psychosis, amotivational syndrome, or medical complications, as commonly believed? Can tolerance, dependence, or a withdrawal syndrome to cannabis be demonstrated? Is THC-Δ-9 the principal active substance in cannabis? Do different preparations have equivalent behavioral and physiological effects when rated as to their THC-Δ-9 content?

The study strategy was a sequential one. The first step was to identify a sample of users as to their drug use and their personal and social characteristics. From a population of noncannabis smokers, controls were chosen for their similarity with the user sample in regard to age, upbringing, refugee origin, and educational characteristics.

Subjects and controls were examined and their psychiatric, medical, psychological, and social characteristics contrasted. Samples of hashish were obtained and analyzed for their content of known cannabis derivatives; and from these data, the daily use of active constituents (chiefly THC-Δ-9) was estimated.

A subsample of the users ($N = 20$) volunteered to smoke hashish, marijuana, denatured marijuana (placebo), and cigarettes with an infusion of pure THC-Δ-9 during five sessions in the research laboratory. Amounts of THC-Δ-9 varied from 0 to 180 mg THC-Δ-9. Behavioral, psychological, psychophysiological, and EEG measures were recorded.

The next experiment defined withdrawal effects to cannabis. Another subsample of active smokers of hashish ($N = 16$) volunteered to be observed for 6 days in a confined hospital setting. They were allowed to smoke marijuana or placebo cigarettes *ad libitum* during two smoking periods each day. Half the group received placebo cigarettes for 3 days followed by

The summary and opinions expressed in this chapter are the sole responsibility of the author, and do not necessarily reflect the views of other editors or authors in this volume.

marijuana cigarettes for 3 days; the other half smoked marijuana for 3 days followed by placebo. Behavioral, psychophysiological, EEG, and psychological measurements were obtained, in addition to subjective self-ratings and number of cigarettes smoked in each group.

POPULATION CHARACTERISTICS

The hashish smokers came largely from immigrant families and resided in a working-class, immigrant section of Athens. Their mean age was 40.7 years, with an average of 23 years of cannabis use which began during their adolescence (17.6 ± 4.1 years). They smoked hashish an average of 2.3 times a day, inhaling 3.13 ± 0.81 mg THC-Δ-9 a day. The men are high-dose users of tobacco, smoking an average of 38.2 ± 17.6 cigarettes a day. Hashish was usually smoked combined with tobacco, and this combination was used in the experimental studies.

In comparisons with the matched nonuser sample, the users were found to have more palpable livers as the principal medical difference. There were no differences on the laboratory tests, including clinical EEG and echoencephalogram.

The user sample was distinguished from the controls in their psychiatric examinations; they had a higher incidence of psychopathy diagnoses but not of other mental illnesses. None of the men exhibited evidence of an organic psychosis, and in extensive psychological tests there were no signs of organic deterioration. The users had more psychiatric care, a higher incidence of imprisonment related and unrelated to cannabis use, different work records, and a lower incidence of military service.

PHARMACOLOGICAL OBSERVATIONS

The cannabis products studied—hashish, marijuana, and the extract THC-Δ-9—are psychoactive when inhaled after combustion. The products pass the blood-brain barrier rapidly, eliciting well-defined CNS effects characterized by enhancement of EEG alpha activity, a slowing of the mean alpha frequency, and a decrease in fast frequencies.

The central effects are accompanied by systemic sympathomimetic release, as seen in an increased heart rate, pupillary dilation, and decreased finger pulse volume. All the cannabis preparations studied exhibit these effects, but their magnitudes are not directly related to the amounts of THC-Δ-9 in the samples. An analysis of the ratios of THC-Δ-9, cannabidiol (CBD), and cannabinol (CBN) in the samples suggest that the higher relative amounts of CBD and CBN in the hashish samples may have antagonized some of the central effects of THC-Δ-9. The psychoactive properties of cannabis materials may be the resultant of complex interactions among the cannabinoid constitutents, and the many constitutents must be assayed in further assessments of cannabis potency.

QUERIES ANSWERED BY THE STUDY

Does Brain Damage Result from Prolonged Cannabis Use?

Many conventional measures of brain function were used, and in none was there evidence of brain damage. The number of abnormalities in the neurological examination and the EEG were similar to those of the control group; echoencephalograms failed to define ventricular shift or dilation; and psychological tests did not show signs of an organic mental syndrome. In their interactive behavior, these men did not exhibit the memory loss, confabulation, disorientation, or confusion ordinarily associated with organic psychoses.

Hashish, marijuana, and THC-Δ-9 each affected the EEG and performance on psychological tests in a characteristic pattern after inhalation. The effects were transient. The EEG effects of marijuana were no longer measurable 4 hr after smoking, although heart rate changes were still observed. These observations suggest that cannabis is psychoactive (i.e., affects brain functions), but the effects are transient and do not produce the accepted signs of brain damage.

For these men, smoking large amounts of cannabis for extended periods did not result in clinical evidence of brain damage, but the number of users examined was small and the men were selected from among functioning and working members in the community. We cannot exclude the possibility that the men represent a resilient residue of a larger group of users—men who may have succumbed to (at present undefined) consequences of cannabis use; who were resident in mental or neurological hospitals or at home; or who failed to volunteer for other reasons. We did inquire of the psychiatric staffs and we examined patient records at the principal mental and neurological hospitals in and near Athens for patients with neurological or psychiatric dysfunction associated with cannabis use; none were identified. We are aware of the weakness inherent in depending on a chart review of patient records, so we cannot exclude the possibility that our sample is biased—although it seems unlikely that many such cases are resident in Athens and not known to the physicians at the principal neurological and psychiatric hospitals.

Is Prolonged Cannabis Use Associated with Psychiatric Disability?

The question of psychiatric disability after prolonged cannibis use is often rephrased: Does cannabis use lead to the development of an organic psychosis, a paranoid-type psychosis, or an amotivational syndrome? As cited above, we found no evidence, either in the psychiatric evaluations or in laboratory tests, of an organic mental syndrome or an organic-type psychosis, either as a chronic mental condition or as an acute episodic reaction to the acute inhalation of cannabis evaluated to contain THC-Δ-9 in amounts up to 180 mg. The diagnosis of a paranoid psychosis was made in three smokers, and considering all the factors in each case it seemed probable that the symptoms were a manifestation of an endogenous type of illness—but the possibility does exist that cannabis use contributed to their disabilities.

The men occasionally describe a "bad trip" accompanied by ideas of reference, feelings of panic and fear, and thoughts of doom. They also report occasional feelings of intense well-being, with thoughts of greatly enhanced physical and mental powers. These episodes are associated with drug use and are reported as transient and occasional. We cannot exclude the possibility that such psychotic reactions occur with a greater frequency in some subjects, particularly under the usual conditions of unregulated and illegal distribution of cannabis substances, whose potency may vary not only in THC-Δ-9 content but in the amounts of other psychoactive cannabinoids and adulterants (62).

A common view of the amotivational syndrome is that cannabis users withdraw from their social and economic responsibilities, fail to perform their assigned duties as heads of households, or fail to work. We found little evidence that cannabis use led to withdrawal, apathy, or indolence although the work records of the users were more irregular than those of the controls; yet the users subjectively reported that hashish improved their work performance, particularly when the work was manual, repetitive, and boring. These men are similar to cannabis users in Jamaica (32,37,166), Costa Rica (28), and India (123a,207) in this regard.

The users did exhibit a higher incidence of psychopathy than the control, nonuser group. They had a higher incidence of arrests and imprisonments, and a lower incidence of satisfactory military service. These findings emphasize their alienation from the native Greek culture, where cannabis is proscribed and tobacco and alcohol accepted. It is unclear if psychopathy is a result of cannabis use, or if cannabis use is a manifestation of a psychological and behavioral profile that allows the men to continue in their antisocial behavior. The users are in frequent conflict with authorities, and this may contribute to their poor assimilation into the legal and social ethos of the country.

Does Tolerance Develop and Are There Defined Symptoms of Withdrawal?

In studies in the United States, occasional users smoking marijuana or hashish containing up to 22.5 mg THC-Δ-9 still evinced the characteristic euphoria and tachycardia of cannabis use. Others found higher doses, up to 40 mg, to be accompanied by illusory sensations, unpleasant feelings, and confused and frightening thoughts (83). In the high-dose administrations reported by Tassinari et al. (185), doses up to 80 mg THC-Δ-9 resulted in cardiovascular collapse, ataxia, hypersomnia, and abnormal motor movements.

In the initial dose-finding studies in these Greek hashish users, we administered doses of marijuana and hashish assayed at less than 60 mg THC-Δ-9. The men characterized the material as poor, and they valued the results very little. Doses greater than 100 mg THC-Δ-9 were evaluated highly, and they smoked up to 180 mg THC-Δ-9 during a single session without discomfort. We believe these observations define a state of tolerance consistent with the reports of similar high-dose usage in the ganja smokers in Jamaica (37,166).

The men report that smoking hashish 2 to 3 times a day is sufficient to maintain their sense of well-being. During a 3-day withdrawal period in the laboratory, we were unable to define a syndrome of withdrawal, but when hashish again became available the subjects smoked an increased number of cigarettes containing hashish.

In subjects who are alcohol or opiate dependent, tolerance and withdrawal symptoms contribute to their sustained drug use. With hashish use the role of tolerance and withdrawal is unclear. Users interpret increases in irritability and tension as withdrawal and institute drug-seeking behavior. When material is again available, greater amounts of hashish are consumed until satiation occurs. When hashish is unavailable, the users have discontinued hashish use for months or even years, returning to it when it is again available. These experiences suggest that tissue changes (tolerance) and withdrawal symptoms serve to sustain hashish use, although their potency may be less than that which sustains alcohol and opiate use.

Experience with hashish must be interpreted in relation to the use of tobacco, for these men use large amounts of tobacco, smoking an average of 38.2 cigarettes a day. Perhaps the smoking of tobacco may satisfy some of the psychological factors which sustain this combined use of hashish and tobacco.

What Are the Medical Consequences of Prolonged Hashish Use?

Our sample of users was small, although their use of hashish was high. In comparison with the nonuser controls, we found signs of an enlarged liver without changes in other systems. The significance of this finding remains obscure, although the use of alcohol was heavier in the men with palpable livers. Because of our sample size, the incidence of any effect occurring in less than 2% of users was probably missed in this study.

However, when these findings are combined with similar reports from Jamaica (37,166) and Costa Rica (34), it is probable that the medical risks of high-dose cannabis use is not greater than, or similar to, the toxicity of tobacco use. The patterns of toxic changes identified with chronic alcohol or opiate use were not observed in these men, and it is improbable that the long term effects of cannabis approach the toxicity of these substances.

DISCUSSION

The findings in these studies are consistent with earlier observations, including the Indian Hemp (207) and LaGuardia Commissions (121); the recent governmental commissions in Great Britain (206), Canada (111), and the United States (134,135); the detailed studies of ganja users in Jamaica (37,166) and cannabis users in Costa Rica (166), India (32), and Egypt (170,171); and chronic dose studies in occasional U.S. users (50,81, 92,93,125–127,129,149). The studies fail to define an inherent toxicity to the nervous system, mental status, or medical complications for long-term cannabis use.

Differences among the studies are seen largely in the incidence of psychopathologic abnormalities. The studies in Egypt (170,171), Thailand (109), and India (32) are particularly divergent in this regard, with an incidence of cannabis psychosis and the amotivational syndrome that exceeds similar estimates in Greece, Jamaica, and Costa Rica.

Another difference among the studies is in the conclusions observers draw with regard to the dangers inherent in cannabis use. We are not impressed that the range of dangers—physical, psychological, and behavioral—ascribed to cannabis use are inherent in the chemical or pharmacological properties of these substances. Smoking cannabis, even in large quantities, seems less dangerous to users or to society than the penalties meted out to users who are judged guilty of violating cannabis proscriptions.

A troublesome question of these data is: Why is hashish smoked? Considering the penalties of its continued use in the present Greek culture, why is it used? The feelings of relaxation, well-being, and sexual adequacy which accompany hashish smoking are important. In some, dysphoric effects may be felt as pleasurable (99). Tolerance and withdrawal symptoms may contribute to continued use. The effect of hashish on work attitude is also contributory. The men ascribe to hashish certain effects that are described in other cultures with the use of tobacco, cocaine, coffee, and khat: enhancement of work performance, stimulation, and provision of a "break" in an otherwise repetitive, dull, and unsatisfying occupation.

Social factors also make a contribution. The men are introduced to hashish use as part of the rites of passage from adolescence to adulthood in their native culture. Perhaps hashish use satisfies the need for companionship and peer group identification, for as a hashish user he is a member of a select group, sharing smoking materials, rituals, dangers and risks—with a feeling of elitism and worth in a culture which may not value his native abilities.

In psychiatric evaluations, these men exhibit a high incidence of personality disorders. These labels signify their behavior as "deviant" in relation to the conventional classification criteria. Yet the psychiatrists do not ascribe the psychopathic behaviors to cannabis use; rather, they believe that personality factors contributed to the continued use of cannabis in an environment that proscribed its use (174). From these possibilities, the continued use of hashish may serve psychological and social needs, and efforts to decrease its use would best be made along psychosocial lines rather than using punitive, legal, or even medical means (166a).

This study in Athens and those in Jamaica and Costa Rica have done much to answer the concerns of a few years ago. Much of the pressure for the study of cannabis has been relieved contemporaneously with the end of the war in Southeast Asia. Cannabis use has either decreased in other countries as well or the reporting methods have changed, since the concern that hashish use was increasing in Europe is muted today. There is also a decrease in governmental and private financial support for studies of cannabis.

The principal limitation of the present studies of long-term users in Greece, Jamaica, and Costa Rica is the small sample size in each study. It is possible that the samples are biased, not reflecting those users who may have suffered the most significant effects. What has happened to subjects who discontinued their use of cannabis? When and why did they do so? Did any subjects die as a result of cannabis use? If the incidence of medical complications is similar to the incidence among tobacco users, larger, prospective studies to define medical consequences are required.

Cannabis inhalation allows substances to reach the brain and cardiovascular systems rapidly (87). The cannabis plant was an important source of medicinals up to the 1930s, and compounds for a variety of medical uses should again be sought, considering the apparent safety of its derivatives. Cannabis substances have direct effects on the cardiovascular system (105,202) and they may have clinical uses in the management of hypertension. Their direct effects on the central nervous system may have clinical usefulness in modifying mental illnesses, particularly in depressive disorders since the EEG effects are those of euphoriants (54,56,57,151,177). The effects on intraocular pressure and pulmonary volume (184) suggest that trials should also be encouraged in glaucoma and asthma. It is probable that the cannabinoids CBD and CBN may reduce the activity of THC-Δ-9, and further studies of the constituents of cannabis and their interaction should be encouraged as sources for compounds with greater physiological specificity. The symptoms of withdrawal remain ill-defined, and prolonged studies are needed—studies with an abstinence of 3–10 days should be considered initially. The evidence of tolerance development in man is indirect (204). The direct studies of tolerance now underway in California may clarify this issue; but if they do not, additional research in long-term users with emphasis on the rate of dissipation of cannabinoids from the blood would be helpful.

The effects of cannabis on chromosomes, sex hormones, and the development of neoplasms are additional issues that have been raised since these studies were undertaken (108,133). These questions reflect the continuing evaluation of the toxicity of cannabis and so long as these issues remain unresolved, their study will be encouraged.

The most important issues regard the social and cultural factors that lead to the use of cannabis and sustain its use. Combined sociological and psychological studies, with attention to the pharmacological factors of tolerance, should be of high priority (203,204). Finally, the use that governments make of cannabis proscription to control their populations requires intensive political and sociological study (166a).

References

1. Abel, E. (1971): Marihuana and memory: Acquisition or retrieval? *Science*, 173:1038–1040.
2. Allentuck, S. (1944): Organic and systemic functions. In *Mayor's Committee on Marihuana, The Marihuana Problem in the City of New York: Sociological Medical, Psychological, and Pharmacological Studies*. Cattell Press, Lancaster, Pa.
3. Allentuck, S., and Bowman, K. M. (1942): The psychiatric aspects of marihuana intoxication. *Am. J. Psychiatry*, 99:248–251.
4. Ames, F. (1958): A clinical and metabolic study of acute intoxication with Cannabis sativa and its role in the model psychoses. *J. Ment. Sci.*, 104:972–999.
5. Asuni, T. (1964): Socio-psychiatric problems of cannabis in Nigeria. *Bull. Narc.*, 16:17–28.
6. Babor, T. F., Mendelson, J. H., Greenberg, I., and Kuehnle, J. C. (1975): Marihuana consumption and tolerance to physiological and subjective effects. *Arch. Gen. Psychiatry*, 32:1548–1552.
7. Baker-Bates, E. T. (1935): A case of Cannabis indica intoxication. *Lancet*, 1:811.
8. Ballas, C. N. (1968): *The Prophetic Delirium of Pythia*. Soteropoulos, Athens.
9. Barratt, E., Beaver, W., White, R., Blakeney, P., and Adams, P. (1972): The effects of the chronic use of marijuana on sleep and perceptual motor performance in humans. In: *Current Research in Marijuana*, edited by M. F. Lewis, pp. 163–193. Academic Press, New York.
10. Beaconsfield, P., Ginsburg, J., and Rainsbury, R. (1972): Marihuana smoking: Cardiovascular effects in man and possible mechanisms. *N. Engl. J. Med.*, 287:209–212.
11. Beaubrun, M. H., and Knight, F. (1973): Psychiatric assessment of 30 chronic users of cannabis and 30 matched controls. *Am. J. Psychiatry*, 130:309–311.
12. Bech, P., Rafaelsen, L., and Rafaelsen, O. J. (1974): Cannabis: A psychopharmacological review. *Dan. Med. Bull.*, 21:106–120.
13. Benabud, A. (1957): Psycho-pathological aspects of the cannabis situation in Morocco: Statistical data for 1956. *Bull. Narc.*, 9:1–16.
14. Bensusan, A. D. (1971): Marihuana withdrawal symptoms (Letter). *Br. Med. J.*, 3:112.
15. Bernstein, J., Becker, D., Babor, T., and Mendelson, J. (1974): Psychological assessments: cardiopulmonary function. In: *The Use of Marijuana, A Psychological and Physiological Inquiry*, edited by J. H. Mendelson, A. M. Rossi, and R. E. Meyer. Plenum Press, New York.
16. Bialos, D. (1970): Adverse marihuana reactions: A critical examination of the literature with selected case material. *Am. J. Psychiatry*, 127:119–123.
17. Boroffka, A. (1966): Mental illness and Indian hemp in Lagos. *East Afr. Med. J.*, 43:377–384.
18. Bowman, M., and Pihl, R. D. (1973): Cannabis: psychological effects of chronic heavy use: A controlled study of intellectual functioning in chronic users of high potency cannabis. *Psychopharmacologia*, 29:159–170.
19. Boyd, E. S., Boyd, E. H., and Brown, L. E. (1971): Effects of the tetrahydrocannabinols on evoked responses in polysensory cortex. *Ann. NY Acad. Sci.*, 191:100–122.
20. Brill, N. A., and Christie, R. L. (1974): Marihuana use and psychosocial adaptation: Follow-up study of a collegiate population. *Arch. Gen. Psychiatry*, 31:713–719.

21. Bromberg, W. (1934): Marijuana intoxication: A clinical study of Cannabis sativa intoxication. *Am. J. Psychiatry*, 91:303–330.
22. Bromberg, W. (1939): Marijuana: A psychiatric study. *JAMA*, 113:4–12.
23. Brunel, R. (1955): Le monachisme errant dans l'Islam. In: *The 1890 Report of the Health Council of Greece on the Effects of Hashish Use. Greek Agriculture*, (Nov), 525–529. Paris.
24. Bull, J. (1971): Cerebral atrophy in young cannabis smokers. *Lancet*, 2:1420.
25. Caldwell, D. F., Meyers, S. A., Domino, E. F., and Merriam, P. E. (1969): Auditory and visual threshold effects of marihuana in man: Addendum. *Percept. Mot. Skills*, 29:754–759.
26. Campbell, A. M. G., Evans, M., Thomson, J. L. G., and Williams, M. J. (1971): Cerebral atrophy in young cannabis smokers. *Lancet*, 2:1219–1224.
27. Campbell, D. R. (1971): The electroencephalogram in cannabis associated psychosis. *Can. Psychiatr. Assoc. J.*, 16:161–165.
28. Carter, W. E., and Doughty, P. L. (1976): Social and cultural aspects of cannabis use in Costa Rica. *Ann. NY Acad. Sci.* 282:2–16.
29. Casswell, S., and Marks, D. (1973): Cannabis induced impairment of performance of a divided attention task. *Nature (Lond.)*, 241:60–61.
30. Chopra, G. S. (1971): Marihuana and adverse psychotic reactions. *Bull. Narc.*, 23:15–22.
31. Chopra, G. S. (1976): Long-term effects of marijuana in chronic users in India compared to chronic users in the western hemisphere: social-psychological aspects of marijuana abuse. *Ann. NY Acad. Sci. (in press)*.
32. Chopra, G. S., and Smith, J. W. (1974): Psychotic reactions following cannabis use in East Indians. *Arch. Gen. Psychiatry*, 30:24–27.
33. Clark, L. D., Hughes, R., and Nakashima, E. N. (1970): Behavioral effects of marihuana: Experimental studies. *Arch. Gen. Psychiatry*, 23:193–198.
34. Coggins, W. J., Swenson, E. W., Dawson, D. W. W., Fernandez-Salaz, A., Hernandez-Bolanos, J., Jiminez-Antellon, F., Solano, J. R., Vinocur, R., and Faerron-Valdez, F. (1976): The health status of chronic heavy cannabis users. *Ann. NY Acad. Sci.* 282:148–161.
35. Cohen, J. (1968): Multiple regression as general data-analytic system. *Psychol. Bull.*, 70:425–443.
36. Cohen, S. (1976): The 94-day marijuana study. *Ann. NY Acad. Sci.* 282:211–220.
37. Comitas, L. (1976): Cannabis and work in Jamaica: A refutation of the amotivational syndrome. *Ann. NY Acad. Sci.* 282:24–32.
38. Couretas, D. (1937): Addicts in the armed forces. In: *Psychiatric Problems in the Army*. Salonica, Greece (Eds. the Greek Medicine).
39. Creutzfeldt, O. D., and Kuhnt, U. (1967): The visual evoked potential: physiological, developmental, and clinical aspects. *Electroencephalogr. Clin. Neurophysiol. (Suppl.)*, 26:29.
40. Cruickshank, E. K. (1976): Physical assessment of 30 chronic users and 30 matched controls. *Ann. NY Acad. Sci.* 282:162–167.
41. Dalton, W. S., Hartz, R., Lemberger, L., Rodda, B. E., and Forney, R. B. (1976): Influence of cannabidiol on delta-9-tetrahydrocannabinol effects. *Clin. Pharmacol. Ther.*, 19:300–309.
42. Darley, C. F., Tinklenberg, J. R., Roth, W. T., and Arkinson, R. C. (1974): The nature of storage deficits and state-dependent retrieval under marihuana. *Psychopharmacologia*, 37:139–149.
43. Deliyannakis, E., Panagopoulos, C., and Hyott, A. (1970): The influence of hashish on human EEG. *Clin. Electroencephalogr.*, 1:128–140.
44. *Diagnostic Statistical Mental Disorders* (1968), 2nd ed. American Psychiatric Association, Washington, D.C.

45. Dohner, V. A. (1972): Motives for drug use: Adult and adolescent. *Psychosomatics*, 8:317–324.
46. Domino, E. F. (1971): Neuropsychopharmacologic studies of marihuana: Some synthetic and natural THC derivatives in animals and man. *Ann. NY Acad. Sci.*, 191:166–191.
47. Domino, E. F., Hardman, H. F., and Seevers, M. H. (1971): Central nervous system action of some synthetic tetrahydrocannabinol derivatives. *Pharmacol. Rev.*, 23:317–336.
48. Dornbush, R., and Kokkevi, A. (1976): The acute effects of various cannabis substances on cognitive, perceptual, and motor performance in very long-term hashish users. In: *Pharmacology of Marihuana*, edited by M. C. Braude and S. Szara, pp. 421–428. Raven Press, New York.
49. Dornbush, R. L. (1974): Marijuana and memory: Effects of smoking on storage. *Trans. NY Acad. Sci.*, 26:94–100.
50. Dornbush, R. L., Clare, G., Zaks, A., Crown, P., Volavka, J., and Fink, M. (1972): 21-Day administration of marijuana in male volunteers. In: *Current Research in Marijuana*, edited by M. Lewis, pp. 115–128. Academic Press, New York.
51. Dornbush, R. L., Fink, M., and Freedman, A. M. (1971): Marihuana, memory, and perception. *Am. J. Psychiatry*, 128:194–198.
51a. Dornbush, R. L., Freedman, A. M. and Fink, M. (1976). *Chronic Cannabis Use. Annals NY Acad. Sci.* Volume 282, 430 pp.
52. Eddy, N., Halbach, H., Isbell, H., and Seevers, M. (1965): Drug dependence: Its significance and characteristics. *Bull. WHO*, 32:721–733.
53. Ferraro, D. P., and Grisham, M. G. (1971): Tolerance to the behaviour effects of marihuana in chimpanzees. *Physiol. Behav.*, 9:49–54.
54. Fink, M. (1969): EEG and human psychopharmacology. *Annu. Rev. Pharmacol.*, 9:241–258.
55. Fink, M. (1973): Effects of cannabis on human EEG and heart rate—evidence of tolerance development on chronic use. In: *Psychopharmacology, Sexual Disorders, and Drug Abuse*, edited by T. A. Ban, J. R. Boissier, G. J. Gjessa, H. Heimann and L. Hollister T. A. Ban et al., pp. 703–704. Avicenum, Prague.
56. Fink, M. (1975): Prediction of clinical activity of drugs in man. In: *Predictiveness in Psychopharmacology: Preclinical and Clinical Correlations*, edited by A. Sudilovsky, S. Gershon, and B. Beer, pp. 65–87, 89–103. Raven Press, New York.
57. Fink, M. (1976): Cerebral effects of acute and chronic inhalation of hashish, marijuana, and TCH-delta-9 in man. *Ann. NY Acad. Sci.* 282:387–398.
58. Fink, M., Volavka, J., Panayiotopoulos, C. P., and Stefanis, C. (1976): Quantitative EEG studies of marijuana, delta-9-tetrahydrocannabinol, and hashish in man. In: *The Pharmacology of Marijuana*, edited by M. C. Braude and S. Szara, pp. 383–391. Raven Press, New York.
59. Ford, R. D., and McMillan, D. E. (1971): Behavioral tolerance and cross-tolerance to 1-delta-8 THC and 1-delta-9 THC in pigeons and rats. *Fed. Proc.*, 30:279.
60. Frank, I. M., Epps, L. D., and Rickles, W. (1973): Psychological and physiological effects of chronic marijuana administration in man. *Psychopharmacol. Bull.*, 9:28–29.
61. Frank, I. M., Lessin, P., Hahn, P., Cohen, S., and Szara, S. (1976): The 94-day marihuana study. In: *Pharmacology of Marihuana*, edited by M. C. Braude and S. Szara, pp. 673–680. Raven Press, New York.
61a. Frazer, J. D. (1949): Withdrawal symptoms in *Cannabis indica* addicts. *Lancet*, 2:747–748.

62. Freedman, A. M., and Fink, M. (1972): Cannabis psychosis. In: *Biochemical and Pharmacologic Aspects of Dependence and Reports on Marijuana Research*, edited by H. M. van Praag, pp. 194–204. Ervin F. Bohn, Amsterdam.

63. Galanter, M., Weingartner, H., Vaughan, T. B., Roth, W. T., and Wyatt, R. J. (1973): Delta-9-transtetrahydrocannabinol and natural marihuana: A controlled comparison. *Arch. Gen. Psychiatry*, 28:278–281.

64. Galanter, M., Wyatt, R. J., Lemberger, L., Weingartner, H., Vaughn, T. B., and Roth, W. J. (1972): Effects on humans of delta-9-tetrahydrocannabinol administered by smoking. *Science*, 176:934–936.

65. Gelpke, R. (1966): *Vom Rausch im Orient und Okzident*. Verlag, Stuttgart.

66. Grant, I., Rochford, J., Fleming, T., and Stunkard, A. (1973): A neuropsychological assessment of the effects of moderate marijuana use. *J. Nerv. Ment. Dis.*, 156:278–280.

67. Grilly, D. M., Ferraro, D. P., and Marriott, R. G. (1973): Long-term interactions of marijuana and behavior in champanzees. *Nature (Lond.)*, 242:119–120.

68. Grinspoon, L. (1971): *Marihuana Reconsidered*. Harvard University Press, Cambridge.

69. Haines, L., and Green, W. (1970): Marihuana use patterns. *Br. J. Addict.*, 65:347–362.

70. Halikas, J. A. (1974): Marijuana use and psychiatric illness. In: *Marijuana: Effects on Human Behavior*, edited by L. L. Miller, pp. 265–299. Academic Press, New York.

71. Halikas, J. A., and Rimmer, J. D. (1974): Predictors of multiple drug abuse. *Arch. Gen. Psychiatry*, 31:414–418.

72. Halikas, J. A., Goodwin, D. W., and Guze, S. B. (1971): Marihuana effects: A survey of regular users. *JAMA*, 217:692–694.

73. Halikas, J. A., Goodwin, D. W., and Guze, S. B. (1972): Marijuana use and psychiatric illness. *Arch. Gen. Psychiatry*, 27:162–165.

74. Hartwich, C. (1911): *Die Menschlichen Genussmittel: Ihre Herkunst, Verbreitung, Geschichte, Bestandteile, Anwendung, und Wirkung*. Tauchnitz, Leipzig.

75. Hekimian, L. J., and Gershon, S. (1968): Characteristics of drug abusers admitted to a psychiatric hospital. *JAMA*, 205:125–130.

75a. Henderson, L., Tennant, F. S., and Guerry, R. (1972): Respiratory manifestations of hashish smoking. *Arch. Otolaryng.*, 95:248–251.

76. Henley, J. R., and Adams, L. D. (1973): Marihuana use in post-collegiate cohorts: Correlates of use, prevalence patterns and factors associated with cessation. *Soc. Probl.*, 20:514–520.

77. Hepler, R. S., and Frank, I. R. (1971): Marihuana smoking and intraocular pressure. *JAMA*, 217:1392.

78. Hepler, R. S., Frank, I. R., and Petrus, R. (1976): Ocular effects of marijuana. In: *Pharmacology of Marihuana*, edited by M. Braude and S. Szara, pp. 815–824. Raven Press, New York.

79. Hochman, J. S., and Brill, N. Q. (1973): Chronic marihuana use and psychosocial adaptation. *Am. J. Psychiatry*, 130:132–140.

79a. Hochman, J. S. and N. Q. Brill. (1971): Chronic marihuana usage and liver function. Lancet II: 818.

80. Hockman, C. H., Perrin, R. G., and Kalant, H. Electroencephalographic and behavioral alterations produced by Δ^1-tetrahydrocannabinol. *Science*, 172:968–970.

81. Hollister, L. E. (1971): Marihuana in man: Three years later. *Science*, 172:21–29.

82. Hollister, L. E., and Gillespie, H. K. (1970): Marihuana, ethanol, and dextroamphetamine: Mood and mental function alterations. *Arch. Gen. Psychiatry*, 23:199–203.

83. Hollister, L. E., Richards, R. K., and Gillespie, H. K. (1968): Comparison of tetrahydrocannabinol and synhexyl in man. *Clin. Pharmacol. Ther.*, 9:783–791.

84. Hosko, M. J., Kochar, M. S., and Wang, R. I. (1973): Effects of orally administered delta-9-tetrahydrocannabinol in man. *Clin. Pharmacol. Ther.*, 14:344–352.

85. Isbell, H., and Jasinski, D. R. (1969): A comparison of LSD-25 with (−)delta-9-transtetrahydrocannabinol (THC) and attempted cross-tolerance between LSD and THC. *Psychopharmacologia*, 14:115–123.

86. Isbell, H., Gorodetzsky, C. W., Jasinski, D., Claussen, U., von Spulak, F., and Korte, F. (1967): Effects of (−)delta-9-transtetrahydrocannabinol in man. *Psychopharmacologia*, 11:184–188.

87. Jaffe, J. H. (1965): Cannabis (marihuana). In: *The Pharmacological Basis of Therapeutics*, edited by L. S. Goodman and A. Gilman, 3rd ed. MacMillan, New York.

88. Jaffe, J. H., and Sharpless, S. K. (1968): Pharmacologic denervation supersensitivity in the central nervous system: a theory of physical dependence. *Proc. Assoc. Res. Nerv. Ment. Dis.*, 46:226–246.

89. Jasinski, D. R., Haertzen, C. A., and Isbell, H. (1971): Review of the effects in man of marijuana and tetrahydrocannabinols on subjective state and physiologic functioning. *Ann. NY Acad. Sci.*, 191:196–205.

90. Johnson, S., and Domino, E. (1971): Some cardiovascular effects of marijuana smoking in normal volunteers. *Clin. Pharmacol. Ther.*, 12:762–768.

91. Jones, R. T. (1971): Tetrahydrocannabinol and the marijuana-induced social "high" or the effects of the mind on marijuana. *Ann. NY Acad. Sci.*, 191:155–165.

92. Jones, R. T., Benowitz, N., and Bachman, J. (1976): Clinical studies of cannabis tolerance and dependence. *Ann. NY Acad. Sci.* 282:221–239.

93. Jones, R. T., and Benowitz, N. (1976): The 30-day trip—clinical studies of cannabis tolerance and dependence. In: *Pharmacology of Marihuana*, edited by M. Braude and S. Szara, pp. 627–642. Raven Press, New York.

94. Jones, R. T., and Stone, G. C. (1970): Psychological studies of marijuana and alcohol in man. *Psychopharmacologia*, 18:108–117.

95. Karniol, I. G., Shirakawa, I., Kasinski, N., Pfeferman, A., and Carlini, E. A. (1974): Cannabidiol interferes with the effects of delta-9-tetrahydrocannabinol in man. *Eur. J. Pharmacol.*, 28:172–177.

96. Kaymakcalan, S. (1972): Physiological dependence on THC in rhesus monkeys. In: *Cannabis and Its Derivatives*, edited by W. D. M. Paton and J. Crown. Oxford University Press, London.

97. Kaymakcalan, S., and Deneau, G. A. (1972): Some pharmacologic properties of synthetic delta-9-tetrahydrocannabinol (THC). *Acta Med. Turc. (Suppl.)*, 1:1–27.

98. Keeler, M. H. (1967): Adverse reaction to marihuana. *Am. J. Psychiatry (Suppl.)*, 124:674–677.

99. Keeler, M. H. (1968): Motivation for marihuana use: A correlate of adverse reaction. *Am. J. Psychiatry*, 125:386–393.

100. Kerim, F. (1930): Les troubles psychiques dus a l'emploi du hashish. *L'Hygiene Ment.*

101. Keup, W. (1970): Psychotic symptoms due to cannabis abuse. *Dis. Nerv. Syst.*, 31:119–126.

101a. Kew, M. C., Bersohn, L., and Siew, S. (1969): Possible Hepatoxicity of Cannabis. *Lancet,* I:578–579.

102. Kiplinger, G. F., Manno, J. E., Rodda, B. E., and Forney, R. B. (1971): Dose-response analysis of the effects of tetrahydrocannabinol in man. *Clin. Pharmacol. Ther.*, 12:650–657.

103. Klintsch, W. (1970): *Learning, Memory, and Conceptual Processes*, pp. 153–157. Wiley, New York.

104. Klonoff, H. (1974): Marijuana and driving in real-life situations. *Science*, 186:317–324.

105. Kochar, M. S., and Hosko, M. J. (1973): Electrocardiographic effects of marihuana. *JAMA*, 225:25–27.

106. Kolansky, H., and Moore, W. T. (1971): Effects of marihuana on adolescents and young adults. *JAMA*, 216:486–492.

107. Kolansky, H., and Moore, W. T. (1972): Toxic effects of chronic marihuana use. *JAMA*, 222:35–41.

108. Kolodny, R. C., Masters, W. H., Kolodner, R. M., and Toro, G. (1974): Depression of plasma testosterone levels after chronic intensive marihuana use. *N. Engl. J. Med.*, 290:872–874.

109. Kroll, P. (1975): Psychoses associated with marijuana use in Thailand. *J. Nerv. Ment. Dis.*, 161:149–156.

110. Kouretas, D. (1937): Drug-abusers in the army. In: *Psychiatric Topics in the Army*, edited by D. Kouretas and F. Scouras. Thessaloniki (Greek language).

111. LeDain, G., Campbell, I. L., Lehmann, H., Stein, J. P., and Bertrand, M. A. (1972): *Cannabis: A Report of the Commission of Inquiry into the Non-Medical Use of Drugs*. Information Canada, Ottawa.

112. Lemberger, L., Axelrod, J., and Kopin, I. J. (1971): Metabolism and disposition of tetrahydrocannabinoids in naive subjects and chronic marijuana users. *Ann. NY Acad. Sci.*, 191:142–154.

113. Lewis, E. G., Dustman, R. E., Peters, B. A., Straight, R. C., and Beck, E. C. (1973): The effects of varying doses of delta-9-tetrahydrocannabinol on the human visual and somatosensory evoked response. *Electroencephalogr. Clin. Neurophysiol.*, 35:347–354.

114. Liakos, A. (1969): Comparison of drug induced pupillary changes in normal and neurotic subjects. *Ph.D. thesis*, London University.

115. Lonnum, A. (1966): The clinical significance of central cerebral ventricular enlargement. Dissert. Universitetsforlaget, Oslo.

116. Low, M., Klonoff, H., and Marcus, A. (1973): The neurophysiological basis of the marijuana experience. *Can. Med. Assoc. J.*, 108:157–165.

116a. Lundergeg, G. D., Adelson, J., Prosnitz, E. H. (1971): Marihuana induced hospitalization. *JAMA*, 215:1121.

117. Manno, J. E., Kiplinger, G. F., Haine, S. E., Bennett, I. F., and Forney, R. B. (1970): Comparative effects of smoking marihuana or placebo on human motor and mental performance. *Clin. Pharmacol. Ther.*, 11:808–815.

118. Manno, J. E., Kiplinger, G. F., Scholz, N., and Forney, R. B. (1970): The influence of alcohol and marihuana on motor and mental performance. *Clin. Pharmacol. Ther.*, 12:202–211.

119. Marcovitz, E., and Myers, H. J. (1944): The marihuana addict in the army. *War Med.*, 6:382–391.

120. Mayer-Gross, W., Slater, E., and Roth, M. (1960): *Clinical Psychiatry*. Cassell, London.

121. Mayor's Committee on Marihuana (1944): *The Marihuana Problem in the City of New York*. Cattell Press, Lancaster, Pa.

122. McGlothlin, W. H., and West, L. J. (1968): The marihuana problem: An overview. *Am. J. Psychiatry*, 125:126–134.

123. McMillan, D. E., Dewey, W. L., and Harris, L. S. (1971): Characteristics of tetrahydrocannabinol tolerance. *Ann. NY Acad. Sci.*, 191:89–99.

123a. Mehndiratta, S. S. and Wig, N. N. (1975): Psychosocial Effects of Longterm Cannabis Use in India. *Drug and Alcohol Dependence,* 1:71–81.

124. Melges, F. T., Tinklenberg, J. R., Hollister, L. E., and Gillespie, H. K. (1970): Marihuana and temporal disintegration. *Science*, 168:1118–1120.

125. Mendelson, J., Babor, T. F., Kuehnle, J. C., Rossi, A. M., Bernstein, J. G., Mello, N. K., and Greenberg, J. (1976): Behavioral and biological concomitants of chronic marijuana smoking by heavy and casual users. *Ann. NY Acad. Sci.* 282:186–210.

126. Mendelson, J. H., Kuehnle, J., Ellingboe, J., and Babor, T. F. (1974): Plasma testosterone levels before, during, and after chronic marihuana smoking. *N. Engl. J. Med.*, 291:1051–1055.

127. Mendelson, J. H., Rossi, A. M., and Meyer, R. E., editors (1974): *The Use of Marihuana, Psychological and Physiological Inquiry.* Plenum Press, New York.

128. Meyer, R. E. (1975): Psychiatric consequences of marihuana use: the state of the evidence. In: *Marijuana and Health Hazards: Methodological Issues in Current Marihuana Research*, edited by J. R. Tinklenberg. Academic Press, New York.

129. Meyer, R. E., Pillard, R. C., Mirin, S. M., Shapiro, L. M., and Fisher, S. (1971): Administration of marihuana to heavy and casual marihuana users. *Am. J. Psychiatry*, 128:198–204.

130. Miras, C. J. (1969): Experience with chronic hashish smokers. In: *Drugs and Youth, Proceedings of the Rutgers Symposium on Drug Abuse*, edited by J. R. Wittenborn, H. Brill, J. P. Smith, and S. A. Wittenborn. Charles C Thomas, Springfield, Ill.

131. Miras, C. J. (1971): Marihuana and hashish. Presented in a lecture at UCLA.

132. Miras, C. J. (1972): Studies on the effects of chronic cannabis administration to man. In: *Cannabis and Its Derivatives*, edited by W. D. M. Paton and J. Crown. Oxford University Press, London.

133. Nahas, G. G., and Greenwood, A. (1974): The first report of the national commission on marihuana (1972): Signal of misunderstanding or exercise in ambiguity. *Bull. NY Acad. Med.*, 50:55–75.

134. National Commission on Marihuana and Drug Abuse, first report (1972): *Marihuana: A Signal of Misunderstanding.* Government Printing Office. Washington, D.C.

135. National Commission on Marihuana and Drug Abuse, second report (1975): *Marihuana and Health.* Government Printing Office, Washington, D. C.

136. Ng, L. K. Y., Lamprecht, F., Williams, R. B., and Kopin, I. J. (1973): Δ-9-Tetrahydrocannabinol and ethanol: Differential effects on sympathetic activity in differing environmental setting. *Science*, 180:1368–1369.

137. Overton, D. A. (1966): State-dependent learning produced by depressants and atropine-like drugs. *Psychopharmacologia*, 10:6–31.

138. Overton, D. A. (1971): State-dependent or "dissociated" learning produced with pentobarbital. In: *Behavioral Analysis of Drug Action*, edited by J. A. Harvey, pp. 59–73. Scott, Foresman & Co., Glenview, Ill.

139. Overton, D. A. (1973): State-dependent learning produced by addicting drugs. In: *Opiate Addiction: Origins and Treatment*, edited by S. Fisher and A. M. Freedman. Winston, Washington, D.C.

140. Panayiotopoulos, C. P., Scarpalezos, S., and Basiakos, L. (1974): The contribution of visual evoked responses in the diagnosis of homonymous hemianopia. *Minerva Med. Grecsi*, 2:190.
141. Papadopoulos, D. N. (1959): *Cannabis*. Athens.
142. Paton, W. D. M., Pertwee, R. G., and Tylden, E. (1973): Clinical aspects of cannabis action. In: *Marijuana: Chemistry, Pharmacology, Metabolism, and Clinical Effects*, edited by R. Mechoulam, pp. 335–365. Academic Press, New York.
143. Pearl, J. H., Domino, E. F., and Rennick, P. (1973): Short-term effects of marijuana smoking on cognitive behavior in experienced male users. *Psychopharmacologia*, 31:13–24.
144. Pentzopoulos, D. (1962): *The Balkan Exchange of Minorities and Its Impact Upon Greece*. Mouton, Paris.
145. Perez-Reyes, M., and Wingfield, M. (1974): Cannabidiol and electroencephalographic epileptic activity. *JAMA*, 230:1635.
146. Perez-Reyes, M., Timmons, H. C., and Lipton, H. A. (1973): A comparison of the pharmacological activity of delta-9-tetrahydrocannabinol and its monohydroxylated metabolites in man. *Experientia*, 29:1009–1010.
147. Perrin, R. G., and Kalant, H. (1971): Electroencephalographic and behavioral alterations produced by D*l*-tetrahydrocannabinol. *Science*, 172:968–970.
148. Petropoulos, E. (1971): *Rebetika Songs*. Chiotelis, Athens.
149. Pillard, R. C. (1970): Medical progress: Marihuana. *N. Engl. J. Med.*, 283:294–303.
150. Pirch, J. H., Cohn, R. A., Barnes, P. R., and Barratt, E. S. (1972): Effects of acute and chronic administration of marijuana extract on the rat electrocorticogram. *Neuropharmacology*, 11:231–240.
151. Pond, D. A. (1948): Psychological effects in depressive patients of the marihuana homologue synhexyl. *J. Neurol. Neurosurg. Psychiatry*, 11:271–279.
152. Pyrros, D. (1832): *Doctor's Textbook*. Navplion, Tobras.
153. Rafaelsen, L., Christrup, H., Bech, P., and Rafaelsen, O. J. (1973): Cannabis and alcohol: Effects on psychological tests. *Nature (Lond.)*, 242:117–118.
154. Rafaelsen, O. J., Bech, P., Christiansen, J., Christrup, H., Nyboe, J., and Rafaelsen, L. (1973): Cannabis and alcohol: Effects on simulated car driving. *Science*, 173:920–923.
155. Rafaelsen, O. J., Bech, P., and Rafaelsen, L. (1973): Simulated car driving influence by cannabis and alcohol. *Pharmakopsychiatry*, 6:71–83.
156. Raven, J. C. (1964): *Matrix 1938 (Progressive Matrices)*. Editions Scientifiques et Psychotechniques, Paris.
157. Raven, J. C. (1965): *Advanced Progressive Matrices, Set I and II*. H. K. Lewis, London.
158. Reininger, W. (1967): Remnants from prehistoric times. In: *The Book of Grass*, edited by G. Andreus. Grove Press, New York.
159. Renault, P. F., Schuster, C. R., Freedman, D. X., Sikic, B., deMello, D., and Halaris, A. (1974): Repeat administration of marihuana smoke to humans. *Arch. Gen. Psychiatry*, 31:95–102.
160. Renault, P. F., Schuster, C. R., Heinrich, R., and Freedman, D. X. (1971): Marihuana: Standardized smoke administration and dose effect curves on heart rate in humans. *Science*, 174:589–591.
161. Rickles, W. H., Cohen, M. J., Whitaker, C. A., and McIntrye, K. E. (1973): Marijuana induced state-dependent verbal learning. *Psychopharmacologia*, 30:349–354.

162. Rodin, E., and Domino, E. F. (1970): Effects of acute marihuana smoking on the EEG. *Electroencephalogr. Clin. Neurophysiol.*, 29:321.
163. Rodin, E. A., Domino, E. F., and Porzak, J. P. (1970): The marijuana induced "social high:" Neurological and electroencephalographic concomitants. *JAMA*, 213:1300–1302.
164. Rossi, A. M., Babor, T., Meyer, R., and Mendelson, J. (1974): Mood states. In: *The Use of Marijuana: A Psychological and Physiological Inquiry*, edited by J. H. Mendelson, A. M. Rossi, and R. E. Meyer, pp. 115–135. Plenum Press, New York.
165. Roth, W. T. (1975): Subjective benefits and drawbacks of marihuana and alcohol. Presented at The Therapeutic Aspects of Marihuana: A Conference at Ailomar, California.
166. Rubin, V., and Comitas, L. (1975): *Ganja in Jamaica: Medical Anthropological Study of Chronic Marihuana Use*. Mouton, The Hague.
166a. Rubin, V. (1975): *Cannabis and Culture*. Mouton, The Hague.
167. Sandis, E. E. (1973): *Refugees and Economic Migrants in Greater Athens*. E.K.K.E., Athens.
168. Satz, P., Fletcher, J. H., and Sutker, L. S. (1976). Neurophysiologic, intellectual, and personality correlates of chronic marijuana use in native Costa Ricans. *Ann. NY Acad. Sci.* 282:266–306.
169. Schwarz, C. J. (1972): Cerebral atrophy in young cannabis smokers. *Lancet*, 1,374.
170. Soueif, M. I. (1971): The use of cannabis in Egypt: A behavioral study. *Bull. Narc.*, 23:17–28.
171. Soueif, M. I. (1967): Hashish consumption in Egypt with special reference to psychosocial aspects. *Bull. Narc.*, 19:1–12.
172. Spencer, D. J. (1971): Cannabis-induced psychosis. *Int. J. Addict.*, 6:323–326.
173. Spitzer, L. R., Fleiss, L. J., Endicott, J., and Cohen, J. (1967): Mental status schedule. *Arch. Gen. Psychiatry*, 16:459–493.
174. Stefanis, C., Liakos, A., Boulougouris, J., Fink, M., and Freedman, A. M. (1976): Chronic hashish use and mental disorder. *Am. J. Psychiatry*, 133:225–227.
175. Stefanis, C., Liakos, A., and Boulougouris, J. (1976): Incidence of Mental Illness in Hashish Users and Controls. In: Chronic Cannabis Use, edited by R. Dornbush, A. M. Freedman and M. Fink. *Ann. NY Acad. Sci.* 282:58–63.
175a. Stefanis, C., Ballas, C., and Madianou, D. (1975): Sociocultural and Epidemiological Aspects of Hashish Use in Greece. In: Cannabis and Culture, edited by V. Rubin, pp. 303–326, Mouton, The Hague.
175b. Steme, J. and C. Ducastaing. (1960). Les Arterites des Cannabis Indica. *Achives des Maladies du Coeur et des Vaisseaux*, 53:143–147.
176. Stillman, R. C., Weingarten, H., Wyatt, R. J., Gillin, C., and Eich, J. (1974): State-dependent (dissociative) effects of marihuana on human memory. *Arch. Gen. Psychiatry*, 31:81–85.
177. Stockings, G. T. (1947): A new euphoriant for depressive mental states. *Br. Med. J.*, 918–922.
178. Stringaris, M. G. (1933): Zur Klinik der Hashchisch psychosen (Nach studien in Griechenland). *Arch. Psychiatr. Nervenkr.*, 100:522–532.
179. Stringaris, M. G. (1939): Die Haschischsucht. Berlin, J. Springer. Reissued 1972, Berlin, Springer-Verlag.
180. Susser, M. (1972): Cerebral atrophy in young cannabis smokers. *Lancet*, 1:41–42.
181. Talbott, J. A., and Teague, J. W. (1969): Marihuana psychosis: Acute toxic psychosis associated with the use of cannabis derivatives. *JAMA*, 210:299–302.

182. Tart, C. T. (1970): Marijuana intoxication: Common experiences. *Nature (Lond.)*, 226:701–704.
183. Tart, C. T. (1971): *On Being Stoned.* Science and Behavior Books, Palo Alto, California.
184. Tashkin, D. P., Shapiro, B. J., and Frank, I. M. (1973): Acute pulmonary physiologic effects of smoked marijuana and oral Δ9-tetrahydrocannabinol in healthy young men. *N. Engl. J. Med.*, 289:336–341.
185. Tassinari, C. A., Ambrosetto, G., and Gastaut, H. (1976): Clinical and polygraphic studies during wakefulness and sleep of high doses of marihuana and delta-9-THC in man. In: *Pharmacology of Marihuana*, edited by M. Braude and S. Szara, pp. 357–375. Raven Press, New York.
186. Tennant, F. S., Preble, M., Prendergast, T. J., and Ventry, P. (1971): Medical manifestations associated with hashish. *JAMA*, 216:1965–1969.
187. Thacore, V. R., and Shukla, S. R. P. (1976): Cannabis psychosis and paranoid schizophrenia. *Arch. Gen. Psychiatry*, 33:383–386.
188. Tinklenberg, J. R., Kopell, B. S., Melges, F. T., and Hollister, L. E. (1972): Marihuana and alcohol: Time production and memory functions. *Arch. Gen. Psychiatry*, 27:812–815.
189. Tinklenberg, J. R., Melges, F. T., Hollister, L. E., and Gillespie, H. K. (1970): Marihuana and immediate memory. *Nature (Lond.)*, 226:1171–1172.
190. Tsaousis, D. G. (1971): *Structure of the Neo-Hellenic Society.* Gutenberg Press, Gutenberg.
191. Tylden, E. (1967): A case for cannabis? *Br. Med. J.*, 3:335.
192. Vamvakaris, M. (1973): *Autobiography.* Athens.
193. Volavka, J., Crown, P., Dornbush, R., Feldstein, S., and Fink, M. (1973): EEG, heart rate, and mood change ("high") after cannabis. *Psychopharmacologia*, 32:11–25.
194. Volavka, J., Dornbush, R., Feldstein, S., Clare, G., Zaks, A., Fink, M., and Freedman, A. M. (1971): Marijuana, EEG, and behavior. *Ann. NY Acad. Sci.*, 191:206–215.
195. Volavka, J., Dornbush, R., Feldstein, S., and Fink, M. (1972): Effects of delta-9-tetrahydrocannabinol on EEG, heart rate, and mood. *Electroencephalogr. Clin. Neurophysiol.*, 33:453.
196. Vouyoucas, C. N. (1971): *Prevention and Repression of the Use of Drugs for Non-Therapeutic Purposes.* Thessaloniki.
197. Walton, R. P. (1938): *Marihuana: American's New Drug Problem.* Lippincott, Philadelphia.
198. Waskow, I. E., Olsson, J. E., Salzman, C., and Katz, M. M. (1970): Psychological effects of tetrahydrocannabinol. *Arch. Gen. Psychiatry*, 22:97–107.
199. Wechsler, D. (1958): *The Measurement and Appraisal of Adult Intelligence*, 4th ed. Williams & Wilkins, Baltimore.
200. Weil, A., Zinberg, N. E., and Nelson, J. M. (1968): Clinical and psychological effects of marihuana use in man. *Science*, 162:1234–1242.
201. Weiss, J. L., Watanabe, A. M., Lemberger, L., Tamarkin, N. R., and Cardon, P. V. (1972): Cardiovascular effects of delta-9-tetrahydrocannabinol in man. *Clin. Pharmacol. Ther.*, 13:671–684.
202. Wendkos, M. H. (1973): Electrocardiographic effects of marihuana (letter). *JAMA*, 226:789–790.
203. Wikler, A. (1970): Clinical and social aspects of marihuana intoxication. *Arch. Gen. Psychiatry*, 23:320–325.
204. Wikler, A. (1976): Aspects of tolerance to and dependence on delta-9-THC. *Ann. NY Acad. Sci.* 282:126–147.

205. Williams, E. G., Himmelsbach, C. K., Wikler, A., Ruble, D. C., and Lloyd, B. J. (1946): Studies on marihuana and pyrahexyl compound. *Public Health Rep.*, 61:1059–1083.
206. Wootton, Lady (1968): *Cannabis. Report by the Advisory Committee on Drug Dependence.* H. M. Stationery Office, London.
207. Young, W. M., chairman (1969): *Report of the Indian Hemp Drugs Commission 1893–94.* Reprinted: *Marijuana Report of the Indian Hemp Drugs Commission 1893–1894.* Thomas Jefferson Publishing Co., Silver Spring, Maryland.
208. Zabathas, E. (1969): *The Greek-Orthodox Migrants from Asia Minor.* Athens.
209. Zimmerman, I. L., and Woo-Sam, J. M. (1973): *Clinical Interpretation of the Wechsler Adult Intelligence Scale.* Grune & Stratton, New York.

Subject Index

Abstinence symptoms, *see* Withdrawal symptoms

Abstinence syndrome, *see* Withdrawal syndrome

Acute inhalation, *see* Acute study

Acute study
  in Athens and New York, 79
  cognitive performance. 69–78
  heart rate, 95–101
  measurements techniques, 104–106
  methods, 21–23, 55–56, 60–61, 64, 71, 79–80, 92, 96, 104–106
  physiological and psychological effects, 95–101
  procedures schedule, 23
  psychophysiological effects, 103–110
  quantitative EEG, 79–89
  results, 34–38, 40–42, 45–47, 50–53, 56–58, 61–62, 65–67, 71–78, 80–89, 94, 97–101, 106–110
  subjective effects, 63–67
  Visual-Evoked Response, 91–94

Ad libitum smoking, 111–119, *see also* Withdrawal study

Age of users and controls, 35

Agitation, 41

Alcohol use
  distribution of, 4
  rating scale, 56
  for withdrawal-symptom relief, 147

Alcoholism, as exclusion criteria, 12

American Psychiatric Association, diagnostic criteria, 50

American users, 79, 100, 135, 145

Amotivational syndrome, 38, 49, 154

Amphetamine use, as exclusion criteria, 12

Amphetamines, 59–60

Anorexia, 147

Anxiety, 147

Appetite increase, 40

Appetite ratings, 148

Arteritis, 55

Assays, cannabinoids, 87

Asthma, 55

Ataxia, 154

Athens University Medical School, 44

Baglamas, 7

Barbiturates, for withdrawal-symptom relief, 147

Barrage-de-signe test
  acute study, 71–73, 75–78

withdrawal study, 28, 124–127, 129–131, 133

Behavior modification and environmental influences, 66

Blood flow, 103
  increased, vs. decreased FPV, 108
  peripheral, 136

Blood pressure, 136, 142, 144

Bouzouki, 7

Bradycardia, 103

Brain damage, 52, 153

Brain syndrome, acute, 49

Bronchitis, 55–57

Canadian Commission of Inquiry into the Non-Medical Use of Drugs, 63, 122

Cannabidiol (CBD)
  one-dose content in cannabis preparations, 87
  and THC-Δ-9
    effects, 75, 87, 100
    interactions, 100, 101

Cannabinoid interaction, 99, 108
  dose-related, 87
  and THC-Δ-9, 108

Cannabinoids, relative amounts in cannabis preparations, 74, 152

Cannabinol (CBN), 87

Cannabis, *see also* Hashish; Marijuana; THC-Δ-9
  clinical uses, 157–158
  effects
    blood flow, 103
    dose-related, 67, 70
    environmental influences, 66
    memory, 69
    measurement of, 69–78
    pleasant, 40–42
    pulmonary, 103
    unpleasant, 40–42
  first mention as narcotic, 5
  hazards, 158
  medical use, 2
  subjective experiences, 39–42

Cannabis fiber, 1

Cannabis preparations
  acute EEG effects, 79–89
  comparative subjective effects, 65
  physiological vs. psychological effects, 95–101
  THC-Δ-9 contents, 22

Cannabis studies, *see also* specific study
    names and places
  methods
    acute study, 21–23, 55–56, 60–61, 64,
      71, 79–80, 92, 96, 104–106
    withdrawal study, 25–31, 112, 123–124,
      136, 148
  pharmacological observations, 152
  population characteristics, 152
  results
    acute study, 34–38, 40–42, 45–47,
      50–53, 56–58, 61–62, 65–67, 71–78,
      80–89, 94, 97–101, 106–110
    withdrawal study, 112–119, 124–133,
      137–145, 148–149
  sample selection, 11–14, 151
  strategy, 151
Cannabis use, *see also* Hashish use;
    Marijuana use
  and brain damage, 153
  in Byzantine empire, 3
  and cerebral atrophy, 43
  chronic
    and cognitive performance, 69–78
    and heart rate, 21, 55, 118, 143
    hepatotoxic effects of, 55–58
    medical effects of, 56–58
    and mental illness, 49–53
    and motor performance, 69–78
    and enlarged liver, 56–57
    and perceptual tests, 69–78
    prolonged reactions, 49
    and respiratory ailments, 55–58
    subjective experiences, 39–42
  and gastrointestinal complaints, 2
  and headache, 2
  history of, 1–9
  in Moslem society, 4
  during Ottoman occupation, 3–4
  and psychosis, 153–154
    and sexual desire, 2
    and sterility, 2
    and tolerance, 25, 100, 121–123, 154, 156
Cannabis users, *see also* Hashish users
  matching, 13
  mentally ill and normal, 46
  selection of, 13–14
Cardiac response, 108
Cardiovascular collapse, 154
Central nervous system (CNS) response, 43,
    49
Cerebral atrophy, 43, 60
Chronic use, *see also* Cannabis use, chronic;
    Hashish use, chronic, defined, 44
Clinical uses, 157–158
Clinical ratings, 28
Cognitive performance, 21, 69–78
Commission of Inquiry into Non-Medical
    Use of Drugs, 111

Comprehension subtest, 45–47
Concentration ability, 43
Consciousness-modifying plants, 2
Constipation ratings, 148
Continuous performance task (CPT), 70
Control subjects, selection of, 13–14
Corneal reflexes, 55, 57
Costa Rican studies, 44, 47, 50, 154, 157

Data processing, 106, 136
Datura stramonium, 2
Depression, 41, 51, 147
Dervish sects, 4
Diagnostic criteria, 50
Digit span, 71, 74
Digit-span performance test, *see* Digit Sym-
    bol Substitution Test
Digit Symbol Substitution test (DSST),
  in acute study, 70–71, 74, 77
  for psychological testing, 45–47
  in withdrawal study, 29, 122, 124, 126–131,
    133
Dizziness, 41
Dose-related effects, 30, 64, 70, 77, 87–88,
    152, 154
Drachma ratings, 97–100, 142
Driving abilities, 40
Drowsiness, 62
Drugs, active
  differences among, 97–98
  vs. placebo effects, 97
Dry mouth, 40

Earaches, 2
Echo-Encephalography, 58–62
Education level of users and controls, 35
Eginition Hospital, University of Athens, 12
Egyptian users, 43
Electrocardiography (ECG), measurement
    technique of, 104–105
Electrodermal activity, 105, 108–110
Electroencephalography (EEG)
  abnormalities, 43
  alpha activity, 81–82, 84, 86, 88–89
  average frequency, 80–82
  beta activity, 81–83, 86–89
  cannabis effects
    dose-related and time-related, 82–83
    marijuana vs. hashish effect, 88
    placebo vs. active preparations, 80–85
    THC-Δ-9 effect, 23
  clinical, 57, 59–62
  computer analysis, 22, 80
    in four-hour postsmoking, 137–138
    materials and methods, 60–61
  drug effects, 100
  and mastura, 98–100
  theta activity, 81–82, 84, 86, 88–89

Emphysema, 56
Employment patterns of users vs. controls, 37
Encephalography
  air, 43, 60
  echo, 58–62
Endocarditis, 55
Euphoria, 40, 154, see also "High"; Subjective experiences

Facial flushing, 136
Facial pallor, 136
Family history of users vs. controls, 36
Fatigue ratings, 148
Finger pulse volumes (FPV), 104–106, 108
  measurement technique, 105
  and postsmoking results, 139, 141, 143–144
Finger tapping tests, 122
Flashbacks, 49
Flatulence ratings, 148
Floating sensation, 40

Galvanic skin response (GSR), 103–106
Ganja, see Cannabis; Hashish; Marijuana
Gastrointestinal complaints, 2
Goal-directed serial alternation task (GDSA), 66, 70
Grip strength, 57

Habituation effect, 144
Hallucinations, 41, 67
Halstead Category test, 122
Hashish, see also Cannabis; Marijuana; THC-Δ-9, 65, 72–78, 81–89, 93, 97–99, 107–109
  cultivation of, 7
  and marijuana cigarettes vs. placebo, 87–88
  medical uses of, 5
Hashish psychosis, 8
Hashish use
  in Dervish sects, 4
  distribution, 4
  first reports, 7
  history, 1–9
  incidence, 18
  initiation, 34–35, 37
  medical adverse effects, 155
  and opium, 43
  punitive and corrective measures for, 9
  reasons for, 34–35, 37, 156
  sociocultural aspects of, 1–9
  Turkish influence, 8
Hashish use, chronic, see also Acute study; Withdrawal study; Cannabis use, chronic
  and concentration ability, 43

and EEG activity, 59–62
and manual dexterity, 43
Hashish users, see also Cannabis users
  characteristics of, 33–38
  and controls, 16–20
    alcohol use, 13
    composition, 15, 33–38
    education, 14
    family history data, 36
    matching, 13, 38
    personal history data, 35, 37
    selection criteria, 13
    socioeconomic status, 14
    and tobacco use, 13
  distribution, 17
  incidence in population, 18
  job levels, 18
  marital status, 19
  and mental illness, 8, 50–53
  occupation, 19
  selection criteria, 11–12
  socioeconomic status, 18
Hashish users, chronic, see also Cannabis users, chronic
  definition, 11
  EEG activity, 59–62
  medical studies, 55–62
Heart rate, 56, 103–106, 108
  and acute inhalation, 21
  CBD blocking effect, 99
  cannabis preparations effect, 95–101
  and drachma rating, 98, 100
  and drug effects, 100
  four-hour postsmoking measurements, 137
  and "high" correlated, 135
  postsmoking, 143
  and THC-Δ-9, 23, 75, 87
Heart-rate response
  mean, 97
  in withdrawal study, 118
Heroin use as exclusion criteria, 12
Hierarchical multiple regression analyses, 80
"High," see also Subject effects; Mastura
  and acute inhalation, 63–67
  defined, 135
  and heart rate, 98–101
  measurement of, 27
  THC-Δ-9 differential effects on, 88
Hyoscyanus albus, 2
Hypersomnia, 154
Hypotension, 147

Illusions, 41
Imprisonment incidence, 36
Impulsivity, 147
Indian Hemp study, 156
Indian study, comparisons with, 154
Insomnia, 41, 147

Intelligence quotients (IQs), 45–46
Iris size vs. pupil size, 105–106
Irritability, 41, 147, 149

Jamaican studies, 33, 42, 44
  comparisons with, 47, 132, 154, 157
  EEG records, 60
  withdrawal study, 132
Jitteriness, 121

Laboratory tests in withdrawal study, 148
LaGuardia Commission study, 156
LeDain Commission, 70
Liver, palpable, 12, 57
LSD use, 59–60, 90
  as exclusion criteria, 12

Mandragora, 2
Manual dexterity, 43
Marijuana intoxication, *see* "High"
Marijuana use, *see also* Cannabis use; Hash-
    ish use
  ad libitum smoking, 111–119
  American, 79
    vs. Jamaican, 42
  casual vs. heavy, in withdrawal study, 25
  CNS response, 49
Marijuana use
  effects
    factors determining, 70
    on memory, 69
    short-term, 79
    vs. hashish, qualitative difference be-
      tween, 75
  Jamaica and Costa Rica, 44
  non-addictive, 147
  North American studies of, 25
  and other cannabis preparations, 65,
    72–78, 81–89, 93, 97–99, 107–109
  and placebo cigarette smoking, 113–115
  and pyrahexyl, 43
  tolerance, 25, 154–155
  and withdrawal study methods, 25–31
Marijuana use, chronic, *see also* Acute
    study; Cannabis use, chronic
  cognitive, perceptual, and motor effects
    of, 69–78
  definition of, 26
Mastura, see "High"
Mastura ratings, 96–99
  and drugs, 100
  and heart rate, 98–101
  in withdrawal, 118, 139
Measurement methods, 69
Medical adverse effects, 155
Medical studies, 55–62, *see also* Acute
    study; Withdrawal study
  alcohol use, 56

methods, 55–56
  physical examinations, 55
  results, 55–57
Memory, 21, 69–70
Mental deterioration, 43
Mental illness
  incidence, 49–53
  vs. normal, 46
  relation to hashish use, 51–52
Mental performance as dose-related, 77–78
Mescaline, 91
Methodology and methodological problems,
  15–16
Military service, users and controls, 36–37
Mood, *see also* "High"; Subjective experi-
    ences, THC-Δ-9/CBD effects, 87
Motor performance, 21
Multiple linear stepwise regressions, 96
Muscular aches, 147

National Commission on Marijuana and Drug
    Abuse, The, 121
National Institutes of Health (NIDA), U.S.,
    22
  marijuana supplied by, 26
Neurological tests, 148
Neuropsychological tests, *see* Psychological
    tests
Neurosis, 51
Nightmares, 41
Number ordination test, 29, 124, 127, 129–
    131, 133
Nystagmus, 55

Opium
  distribution of use, 4
  and hashish, positive correlation between,
    43
Organic mental syndrome, 62

Palpitations, 41
Panic attack, 41, 49, 64
Paranoia, 50–51
Perceptual performance, 21, 40
Performance impairment as dose-related, 70
Peripheral vasodilation, 136
Persecutory delusions, 41, 67
Personal history, users and controls, 36–37
Personality disorders, 50–53
Perspiration, 147
Pharmacological summary, 152
Photophobia, 147
Physical examination, 55
Physiological effects, and psychological ef-
    fects intercorrelated, 95–101, *see also*
    Heart rate
Piloerection, 147

Placebo
  and active drugs, 80–85, 97
  effects, 131, 149
Plethysmography, 103–106, 136
Pneumoencephalograms, 43, 60
Population characteristics, 152
Post hoc t-tests, 71, 85, 94, 96, 106–107
Postsmoking, *see also* Withdrawal study
  EEG data and VERs, 137–138
  evaluation, 71–78
  heart-rate results, 137
  immediate vs. four-hour measurements, 131, 144–145
Practice effect, 75, 122
Price, *see* Drachma ratings
Problem-solving improvement, 40
Progressive Matrices (PM), 44–47
Psilocybin, 91
Psychedelic drugs, 91
Psychiatric disorders, incidence of, 51–53
Psychiatric interview, 148
Psychiatric treatment, previous, users and controls, 36–37
Psychological effects, *see also* Subjective experiences; Mastura ratings; "High" and physiological effects intercorrelated, 95–101
Psychological tests
  behavior during, 44–45
  characteristics, 43–47
  results, 45–47
  in withdrawal, 28–29, 121–133
Psychopathology score, 148
Psychophysiological effects, 103–110, 135–145
Psychosis, 49–52, 147, 153–154
Pulmonary fibrositis, 55
Pulse rate, *see* Heart rate
Pupil size, 103–108, 110, 136
  four-hour postsmoking, 139
  measurement technique, 105
  and THC-Δ-9, 108
Pyrahexyl
  dosage in withdrawal study, 111
  and marijuana, 43
  withdrawal effects, 147

Rating scales, 148
Raven Progressive Matrices, *see* Progressive Matrices
Rebetiko music, 8
Recollection, 40, *see also* Memory
Relaxation, 40
Respiration, measurement, 105
Respiratory ailments, incidence, 55–58
Respiratory rate, 103, 107
  postsmoking, 139–140
  and THC-Δ-9, 107
  unchanged by cannabis, 136

Restlessness, 147

Sample selection, 11–20, 151
Schizophrenic disorders, 50–52, 60
Seashore Rhythm test, 122
Serial sevens test
  acute studies, 71, 74, 76–77
  withdrawal studies, 28, 124–126, 129, 133
Sexual desire, 2, 40
Similarities subtest, 45–47
Skin conductance level (SCL), 104, 110
Skin conductance response (SCR), 104, 109
Sociocultural aspects of use, 1–9
Solanaceae, 2
Soma, 2
Somatosensory evoked responses, 91
Star tracing, 71, 75, 77
State-dependent effects, 132
Sterility, 2
"Stoned," *see* "High"
Studies; *see also* specific names and places
  methodology, 15–16
Subjective experiences, *see also* "High"; *Mastura* ratings
  acute inhalation, 63–67
  CBD effects, 99
  differential, from cannabis preparations, 95, 97–101
  Jamaican and American users, 132
Superiority feelings, 40
Sweating, 41, 147
Sympathomimetic release, 108

Tachycardia, 108, 110, 154
Tactical performance test, 122
Talkativeness, 40
Tekedes, 8
Temperature, 103–106, 136
  and THC-Δ-9, 107
  measurement, 105
  postsmoking, 139, 141, 143–144
Tendon reflexes, 57
THC-Δ-9
  and CBD, 75, 87, 99, 100
  content
    in cannabis preparations, 22
    in Greek hashish and American marijuana, 37
    in marijuana single-dose, 21
    in NIDA marijuana, 26
  dose-related responses, 30, 64
  effects, 23, 65, 72–78, 81–89, 93, 97–99, 107–109
    central, 152
    on "high", 88
    on VERs, 91–94
  and heart rate, 23, 75, 87
  high-dose results, 154
  interaction with CBD, 101

THC-Δ-9 (*contd.*)
  and *mastura,* 88
  and mental performances, 77
  metabolism, 119
  stimulant effect of, 94
Thought processes, 41
Time-estimation ability, 29, 71, 73, 77, 124, 126, 128, 130
Time sense, 69–70
Tobacco and hashish use, 155
Tolerance, 25, 100, 121–122, 123, 154, 156
Toxic delirium, *see* Brain syndrome
Trail making tests, 122
Tremor, 55, 145
Turkish influence on hashish use, 8

University of Athens, 12
Uvular edema, 56

Vertigo, 57
Visual evoked responses (VERs), 91–94
  amplitude-measurement method, 92
  in postsmoking/withdrawal study, 138
Vomiting, 41

Wechsler Adult Intelligence Scale (WAIS), 44–47, 71

Well-being, sense of, 64
Withdrawal study
  amounts smoked, 111–119
  clinical and laboratory tests, 147–149
  clinical ratings, 28
  first-smoking results, 115–117
  heart-rate, 118, 137, 143
  mastura ratings, 118
  methods and procedures, 25–31, 112, 123–124, 136, 148
  physiological and subjective measurements, 29
  postsmoking measurements, 124–144
  psychological tests, 28–29, 121–133
  psychophysiological changes, 135–145
  results, 112–119, 124–133, 133–145, 148–149
  second-smoking results, 115–117
  smoking format, 27
  smoking session, 115–117
  state-dependent effects, 132
  testing schedule, 28
Withdrawal symptoms, 111, 121, 144, 147
Work performance, 40–41

Yawning, 147

Author Index

The number in parentheses is the citation number; the page numbers where the citation appears precede the parentheses. Italics indicate the page in the reference section (pages 159-169) where the full citation appears.

Abel, E., 21, 30, 70, 83, *159* (1)
Adams, L. D., 37, *162* (76)
Adams, P., 70, *159* (9)
Adelson, J., 55, *164* (116a)
Allentuck, S., 30, 55, 95, *159* (2); 30, 103, 110, *159* (3)
Ambrosetto, G., 42, 89, 92, 94, 154, *168* (185)
Ames, F., 55, 58, 66, 79, 83, 103, 110, 136, *159* (4)
Arkinson, R. C., 70, *160* (42)
Asuni, T., 49, *159* (5)
Axelrod, J., 119, *164* (112)

Babor, T. F., 64, *159* (6); 55, 58, 95, *159* (15); 89, 156, *165* (125); 25, 111, 135, 156, *165* (126); 39, 42, 95, *167* (164)
Bachman, J., 103, 111, 144, 156, *163* (92)
Baker-Bates, E. T., 103, 110, *159* (7)
Ballas, C., 2, *159* (8); 1, *167* (175a)
Barnes, P. R., 79, *166* (150)
Barratt, E., 70, *159* (9); 79, *166* (150)
Basiakos, L., *166* (140)
Beaconsfield, P., 103, 110, 136, 145, *159* (10)
Beaubrun, M. H., 11, 25, 38, 50, 112, *159* (11)
Beaver, W., 70, *159* (9)
Bech, P., 39, 63, 69, 70, *159* (12); *166* (153); *166* (154); 70, *166* (155)
Beck, E. C., 91, *164* (113)
Becker, D., 55, 58, 95, *159* (15)
Benabud, A., 11, 49, *159* (13)
Bennett, I. F., 69, *164* (117)
Benowitz, N., 103, 111, 144, 156, *163* (92); 89, 119, 135, 147, 156, *163* (93)
Bensusan, A. D., 119, 147, *159* (14)
Bernstein, J. G., 55, 58, 95, *159* (15); 89, 156, *165* (125)
Bersohn, L., 55, *164* (101a)
Bertrand, M. A., 25, 26, 63, 64, 70, 95, 111, 122, 135, 156, *164* (111)
Bialos, D., 39, *159* (16)
Blakeney, P., 70, *159* (9)
Boroffka, A., 11, 49, *159* (17)
Boulougouris, J., 52, 157, *167* (174); 25, *167* (175)
Bowman, K. M., 30, 103, 110, *159* (3)
Bowman, M., 44, 132, *159* (18)
Boyd, E. H., 94, *159* (19)

Boyd, E. S., 94, *159* (19)
Brill, N. A., 11, 33, *159* (20)
Brill, N. Q., 33, 44, 50, *162* (79); 58, *162* (79a)
Bromberg, W., 39, *160* (21); 42, 119, *160* (22)
Brown, L. E., 94, *159* (19)
Brunel, R., 4, *160* (23)
Bull, J., 60, *160* (24)

Caldwell, D. F., 70, 111, *160* (25)
Campbell, A. M. G., 43, 57, 60, *160* (26)
Campbell, D. R., 43, 59, *160* (27)
Campbell, I. L., 25, 26, 63, 64, 70, 95, 111, 122, 135, 156, *164* (111)
Cardon, P. V., 145, *168* (201)
Carlini, E. A., 69, 75, 87, 88, 99, *163* (95)
Carter, W. E., 154, *160* (28)
Casswell, S., 69, 70, *160* (29)
Chopra, G. S., 11, 33, 49, *160* (30); 43, *160* (31); 154, 156, *160* (32)
Christiansen, J., *166* (154)
Christie, R. L., 11, 33, 159 (20)
Christrup, H., *166* (153); *166* (154)
Clare, G., 25, 64, 69, 70, 86, 89, 95, 96, 103, 108, 119, 122, 135, 156, *161* (50); 79, 80, 86, 95, 99, 135, 136, *168* (194)
Clark, L. D., 21, 69, *160* (33)
Claussen, U., 66, 95, 103, 110, 136, *163* (86)
Coggins, W. J., 50, 112, 155, *160* (34)
Cohen, J., 22, 80, 96, *160* (35); 29, *167* (173)
Cohen, M. J., 103, 110, *166* (161)
Cohen, S., 89, 149, *160* (36); 95, 119, *161* (61)
Cohn, R. A., 79, *166* (150)
Comitas, L., 154, 155, 156, *160* (37); 33, 42, 59, 60, 112, 132, 154, 155, 156, *167* (166)
Couretas, D., 8, 57, *160* (38)
Creutzfeldt, O. D., *160* (39)
Crown, P., 25, 64, 69, 70, 86, 89, 95, 96, 103, 108, 119, 122, 135, 156, *161* (50); 21, 64, 67, 79, 80, 86, 95, 100, 108, 135, *168* (193)
Cruickshank, E. K., *160* (40)

Dalton, W. S., 87, *160* (41)
Darley, C. F., 70, *160* (42)
Dawson, W. W., 50, 112, 155, *160* (34)
Deliyannakis, E., 59, 79, *160* (43)
deMello, D., 21, 25, 123, 135, *166* (159)
Deneau, G. A., 121, *163* (97)

Dewey, W. L., 121, *165* (123)
Diagnostic Statistical Mental Disorders, 50, *160* (44)
Dohner, V. A., 37, *161* (45)
Domino, E. F., 70, 111, *160* (25); 21, 94, 103, 110, *161* (46); 21, 94, 110, *161* (47); 21, 103, 108, *163* (90); 69, *166* (143); 55, 79, 86, 91, 111, 135, *167* (162); 79, 86, 91, 135, *167* (163)
Dornbush, R., 69, 123, *161* (48); 21, 44, *161* (49); 25, 64, 69, 70, 86, 89, 95, 96, 103, 108, 119, 122, 135, 156, *161* (50); 21, 69, 70, 79, 135, *161* (51); *161* (51a); 21, 64, 67, 79, 80, 86, 95, 100, 108, 135, *168* (193); 79, 80, 86, 95, 99, 135, 136, *168* (194); 80, 95, *168* (195)
Doughty, P. L., 154, *160* (28)
Ducastaing, C., 55, *167* (175b)
Dustman, R. E., 91, *164* (113)

Eddy, N., 101, *161* (52)
Eich, J., 132, *167* (176)
Ellingboe, J., 25, 111, 135, 156, *165* (126)
Endicott, J., 29, *167* (173)
Epps, L. D., 103, 105, 106, 122, *161* (60)
Evans, M., 43, 57, 60, *160* (26)

Faerron-Valdez, F., 50, 112, 155, *160* (34)
Feldstein, S., 21, 64, 67, 79, 80, 86, 95, 100, 108, 135, *168* (193); 79, 80, 86, 95, 99, 135, 136, *168* (194); 80, 95, *168* (195)
Fernandez-Salaz, A., 50, 112, 155, *160* (34)
Ferraro, D. P., 121, *161* (53); 121, *162* (67)
Fink, M., 25, 64, 69, 70, 86, 89, 95, 96, 103, 108, 119, 122, 135, 156, *161* (50); 21, 69, 70, 79, 135, *161* (51); *161* (51a); 79, 157, *161* (54); 79, 86, *161* (55); 79, 157, *161* (56); 43, 86, 157, *161* (57); 43, 86, *161* (58); 49, 154, *162* (62); 52, 157, *167* (174); 21, 64, 67, 79, 80, 86, 95, 100, 108, 135, *168* (193); 79, 80, 86, 95, 99, 135, 136, *168* (194); 80, 95, *168* (195)
Fisher, S., 39, 70, 95, 156, *165* (129)
Fleiss, L. J., 29, *167* (173)
Fleming, T., 25, 43, *162* (66)
Fletcher, J. H., 44, 47, *167* (168)
Ford, R. D., 121, *161* (59)
Forney, R. B., 87, *160* (41); 70, 103, 108, *164* (102); 69, *164* (117); *164* (118)
Frank, I. M., 103, 105, 106, 122, *161* (60); 95, 119, *161* (61); 157, *168* (184)
Frank, I. R., 103, *162* (77); 103, *162* (78)
Frazer, J. D., 147, *161* (61a)
Freedman, A. M., 21, 69, 70, 79, 135, *161* (51); *161* (51a); 49, 154, *162* (62); 52, 157, *167* (174); 79, 80, 86, 95, 99, 135, 136, *168* (194)

Freedman, D. X., 21, 25, 123, 135, *166* (159); 21, 25, 123, 135, *166* (160)

Galanter, M., 79, *162* (63); 95, 100, 162 (64)
Gastaut, H., 42, 89, 92, 94, 154, *168* (185)
Gelpke, R., 4, *162* (65)
Gershon, S., 39, 42, 83, *162* (75)
Gillespie, H. K., 70, 135, *163* (82); 39, 103, 108, *163* (83); 64, 66, 70, *165* (124); 21, 70, *168* (189)
Gillin, C., 132, *167* (176)
Ginsburg, J., 103, 110, 136, 145, *159* (10)
Goodwin, D. W., 33, 42, 64, *162* (72); 11, 33, 52, *162* (73)
Gorodetzsky, C. W., 66, 95, 103, 110, 136, *163* (86)
Grant, I., 25, 43, *162* (66)
Green, W., 39, *162* (69)
Greenberg, I., 64, *159* (6)
Greenberg, J., 89, 156, *165* (125)
Greenwood, A., 157, *165* (133)
Grilly, D. M., 121, *162* (67)
Grinspoon, L., 39, 63, 147, *162* (68)
Grisham, M. G., 121, *161* (53)
Guerry, R., 55, *162* (75a)
Guze, S. B., 33, 42, 64, *162* (72); 11, 33, 52, *162* (73)

Haertzen, C. A., 135, *163* (89)
Hahn, P., 95, 119, *161* (61)
Haine, S. E., 69, *164* (117)
Haines, L., 39, *162* (69)
Halaris, A., 21, 25, 123, 135, *166* (159)
Halbach, H., 101, *161* (52)
Halikas, J. A., 49, 50, *162* (70); 33, *162* (71); 33, 42, 64, *162* (72); 11, 33, 52, *162* (73)
Hardman, H. F., 29, 94, 110, *161* (47)
Harris, L. S., 121, *165* (123)
Hartwich, C., 2, *162* (74)
Hartz, R., 87, *160* (41)
Heinrich, R., 95, 103, 135, *166* (160)
Hekimian, L. J., 39, 42, 83, *162* (75)
Henderson, L., 55, *162* (75a)
Henley, J. R., 37, *162* (76)
Hepler, R. S., 103, *162* (77); 103, *162* (78)
Hernandez-Bolanos, J., 50, 112, 155, *160* (34)
Himmelsbach, C. K., 25, 43, 79, 96, 103, 111, 121, 123, 135, 147, *169* (205)
Hochman, J. S., 33, 44, 50, *162* (79); 58, *162* (79a)
Hockman, C. H., 79, *162* (80)
Hollister, L. E., 63, 66, 89, 95, 99, 136, 156, *162* (81); 70, 135, *163* (82); 39, 103, 108, *163* (83); 64, 66, 70, *165* (124); 21, 69, 91, 94, *168* (188); 21, 70, *168* (189)
Hosko, M. J., 69, 70, 145, *163* (84); 157, *164* (105)

Hughes, R., 21, 69, *160* (33)
Hyott, A., 59, 79, *160* (43)

Isbell, H., 101, *161* (52); 103, 136, 145, *163* (85); 66, 95, 103, 110, 136, *163* (86); 135, *163* (89)

Jaffe, J. H., 108, 157, *163* (87); 119, *163* (88)
Jasinski, D. R., 103, 136, 145, *163* (85); 66, 95, 103, 110, 136, *163* (86); 135, *163* (89)
Jiminez-Antellon, F., 50, 112, 155, *160* (34)
Johnson, S., 21, 103, 108, *163* (90)
Jones, R. T., 25, 63, 64, 67, 147, *163* (91); 103, 111, 144, 156, *163* (92); 89, 119, 135, 147, 156, *163* (93); 69, 70, 79, *163* (94)

Kalant, H., 79, *162* (80); 103, *166* (147)
Karniol, I. G., 69, 75, 87, 88, 99, *163* (95)
Kasinski, N., 69, 75, 87, 88, 99, *163* (95)
Katz, M. M., 30, 70, 103, *168* (198)
Kaymakcalan, S., 121, 147, *163* (96); 121, *163* (97)
Keeler, M. H., 33, 39, 42, *163* (98); 39, 42, 156, *163* (99)
Kerim, F., 5, *163* (100)
Keup, W., 49, *163* (101)
Kew, M. C., 55, *164* (101a)
Kiplinger, G. F., 70, 103, 108, *164* (102); 69, *164* (117); *164* (118)
Klintsch, W., 69, *164* (103)
Klonoff, H., 103, 136, *164* (116); *164* (104)
Knight, F., 11, 25, 38, 50, 112, *159* (11)
Kochar, M. S., 69, 70, 145, *163* (84); 157, *164* (105)
Kokkevi, A., 69, 123, *161* (48)
Kolansky, H., 43, 49, *164* (106); 11, 42, 49, *164* (107)
Kolodner, R. M., 157, *164* (108)
Kolodny, R. C., 157, *164* (108)
Kopell, B. S., 21, 69, 91, 94, *168* (188)
Kopin, I. J., 119, *164* (112); 108, *165* (136)
Kouretas, D., 6, 7, *164* (110)
Kroll, P., 156, *164* (109)
Kuehnle, J. C., 64, *159* (6); 89, 156, *165* (125); 25, 111, 135, 156, *165* (126)
Kuhnt, U., *160* (39)

Lamprecht, F., 108, *165* (136)
LeDain, G., 25, 26, 63, 64, 70, 95, 111, 122, 135, 156, *164* (111)
Lehmann, H., 25, 26, 63, 64, 70, 95, 111, 122, 135, 156, *164* (111)
Lemberger, L., 87, *160* (41); 95, 100, *162* (64); 119, *164* (112); 145, *168* (201)
Lessin, P., 95, 119, *161* (61)
Lewis, E. G., 91, *164* (113)
Liakos, A., 105, *164* (114); 52, 157, *167* (174); 25, *167* (175)

Lipton, H. A., 103, *166* (146)
Lloyd, B. J., 25, 43, 79, 96, 103, 111, 121, 123, 135, 147, *169* (205)
Lonnum, A., 62, *164* (115)
Low, M., 103, 136, *164* (116)
Lundergeg, G. D., 55, *164* (116a)

Madianou, D., 1, *167* (175a)
Manno, J. E., 70, 103, 108, *164* (102); 69, *164* (117); *164* (118)
Marcovitz, E., 66, *164* (119)
Marcus, A., 103, 136, *164* (116)
Marks, D., 69, 70, *160* (29)
Marriott, R. G., 121, *162* (67)
Masters, W. H., 157, *164* (108)
Mayer-Gross, W., 33, 50, *164* (120)
Mayor's Committee on Marihuana, 39, 156, *164* (121)
McGlothlin, W. H., 38, 147, *165* (122)
McIntyre, K. E., 103, 110, *166* (161)
McMillan, D. E., 121, *161* (59); 121, *165* (123)
Mehndiratta, S. S., 154, *165* (123a)
Melges, F. T., 64, 66, 70, *165* (124); 21, 69, 91, 94, *168* (188); 21, 70, *168* (189)
Mello, N. K., 89, 156, *165* (125)
Mendelson, J. H., 64, *159* (6); 55, 58, 95, *159* (15); 89, 156, *165* (125); 25, 111, 135, 156, *165* (126); 63, 95, 119, 135, 149, 156, *165* (127); 39, 42, 95, *167* (164)
Merriam, P. E., 70, 111, *160* (25)
Meyer, R. E., 63, 95, 119, 135, 149, 156, *165* (127); 49, *165* (128); 39, 70, 95, 156, 165, (129); 39, 42, 95, *167* (164)
Meyers, S. A., 70, 111, *160* (25)
Mirin, S. M., 39, 70, 95, 156, *165* (129)
Miras, C. J., 43, 59, 79, *165* (130); *165* (131); *165* (132)
Moore, W. T., 43, 49, *164* (106); 11, 42, 49, *164* (107)
Myers, H. J., 66, *164* (119)

Nahas, G. G., 157, *165* (133)
Nakashima, E. N., 21, 69, *160* (33)
National Commission on Marihuana and Drug Abuse, 1st report, 21, 26, 121, 122, 156, *165* (134)
National Commission on Marihuana and Drug Abuse, 2nd report, 49, 156, *165* (135)
Nelson, J. M., 25, 37, 42, 63, 69, 70, 103, 110, 132, 135, 145, *168* (200)
Ng, L. K. Y., 108, *165* (136)
Nyboe, J., *166* (154)

Olsson, J. E., 39, 70, 103, *168* (198)
Overton, D. A., 132, *165* (137); 132, *165* (138); 132, *165* (139)

Panagopoulos, C., 59, 79, *160* (43)
Panayiotopoulos, C. P., 43, 86, *161* (58); *166* (140)
Papadopoulos, D. N., 1, 2, 6, 8, *166* (141)
Paton, W. D. M., 135, 147, *166* (142)
Pearl, J. H., 69, *166* (143)
Pentzopoulos, D., 4, *166* (144)
Perez-Reyes, M., 25, 63, 119, 122, *166* (145); 103, *166* (146)
Perrin, R. G., 79, *162* (80); 103, *166* (147)
Pertwee, R. G., 135, 147, *166* (142)
Peters, B. A., 91, *164* (113)
Petropoulos, E., 7, 8, *166* (148)
Petrus, R., 103, *162* (78)
Pfeferman, A., 69, 75, 87, 88, 99, *163* (95)
Pihl, R. D., 44, 132, *159* (18)
Pillard, R. C., 39, 70, 95, 156, *165* (129); 156, *166* (149)
Pirch, J. H., 79, *166* (150)
Pond, D. A., 157, *166* (151)
Porzak, J. P., 79, 86, 91, 135, *167* (163)
Preble, M., *168* (186)
Prendergast, T. J., *168* (186)
Prosnitz, E. H., 55, *164* (116a)
Pyrros, D., 5, *166* (152)

Rafaelsen, L., 39, 63, 69, 70, *159* (12); *166* (153); *166* (154); 70, *166* (155)
Rafaelsen, O. J., 39, 63, 69, 70, *159* (12); *166* (153); *166* (154); 70, *166* (155)
Rainsbury, R., 103, 110, 136, 145, *159* (10)
Raven, J. C., 44, *166* (156); 44, *166* (157)
Reininger, W., 1, 3, *166* (158)
Renault, P. F., 21, 25, 123, 135, *166* (159); 95, 103, 135, *166* (160)
Rennick, P., 69, *166* (143)
Richards, R. K., 39, 103, 108, *163* (83)
Rickles, W., 103, 105, 106, 122, *161* (60); 103, 110, *166* (161)
Rimmer, J. D., 33, *162* (71)
Rochford, J., 25, 43, *162* (66)
Rodda, B. E., 87, *160* (41); 70, 103, 108, *164* (102)
Rodin, E., 55, 79, 86, 91, 111, 135, *167* (162); 79, 86, 91, 135, *167* (163)
Rossi, A. M., 89, 156, *165* (125); 63, 95, 119, 135, 149, 156, *165* (127); 39, 42, 95, *167* (164)
Roth, M., 33, 50, *164* (120)
Roth, W. J., 95, 100, *162* (64)
Roth, W. T., 70, *160* (42); 79, *162* (63); 39, 42, 63, 64, 132, *167* (165)
Rubin, V., 33, 42, 59, 60, 112, 132, 154, 155, 156, *167* (166); 157, 158, *167* (166a)
Ruble, D. C., 25, 43, 79, 96, 103, 111, 121, 123, 135, 147, *169* (205)

Salzman, C., 30, 70, 103, *168* (198)
Sandis, E. E., 5, 19, *167* (167)

Satz, P., 44, 47, *167* (168)
Scarpalezos, S., *166* (140)
Scholz, N., *164* (118)
Schuster, C. R., 21, 25, 123, 135, *166* (159); 95, 103, 135, *166* (160)
Schwarz, C. J., 60, *167* (169)
Seevers, M., 29, 94, 110, *161* (47); 101, *161* (52)
Shapiro, B. J., 157, *168* (184)
Shapiro, L. M., 39, 70, 95, 156, *165* (129)
Sharpless, S. K., 119, *163* (88)
Shirakawa, I., 69, 75, 87, 88, 99, *163* (95)
Shukla, S. R. P., 42, 69, *168* (187)
Siew, S., 55, *164* (101a)
Sikic, B., 21, 25, 123, 135, *166* (159)
Slater, E., 33, 50, *164* (120)
Smith, J. W., 156, *160* (32)
Solano, J. R., 50, 112, 155, *160* (34)
Soueif, M. I., 43, 156, *167* (170); 37, 156, *167* (171)
Spencer, D. J., 42, *167* (172)
Spitzer, L. R., 29, *167* (173)
von Spulak, F., 66, 95, 103, 110, 136, *163* (86)
Stefanis, C., 43, 86, *161* (58); 52, 157, *167* (174); 25, *167* (175); 1, *167* (175a)
Stein, J. P., 25, 26, 63, 64, 70, 95, 111, 122, 135, 156, *164* (111)
Steme, J., 55, *167* (175b)
Stillman, R. C., 132, *167* (176)
Stockings, G. T., 157, *167* (177)
Stone, G. C., 69, 70, 79, *163* (94)
Straight, R. C., 91, *164* (113)
Stringaris, M. G., 8, 49, *167* (178); 4, 6, 7, 8, *167* (179)
Stunkard, A., 25, 43, *162* (66)
Susser, M., 60, *167* (180)
Sutker, L. S., 44, 47, *167* (168)
Swenson, E. W., 50, 112, 155, *160* (34)
Szara, S., 95, 119, *161* (61)

Talbott, J. A., 66, *167* (181)
Tamarkin, N. R., 145, *168* (201)
Tart, C. T., 42, 64, *168* (182); 39, *168* (183)
Tashkin, D. P., 157, *168* (184)
Tassinari, C. A., 42, 89, 92, 94, 154, *168* (185)
Teague, J. W., 66, *167* (181)
Tennant, F. S., 55, *162* (75a); *168* (186)
Thacore, V. R., 42, 69, *168* (187)
Thomson, J. L. G., 43, 57, 60, *160* (26)
Timmons, H. C., 103, *166* (146)
Tinklenberg, J. R., 70, *160* (42); 64, 66, 70, *165* (124); 21, 69, 91, 94, *168* (188); 21, 70, *168* (189)
Toro, G., 157, *164* (108)
Tsaousis, D. C., 5, *168* (190)
Tylden, E., 135, 147, *166* (142); 66, *168* (191)

Vamvakaris, M., 7, *168* (192)
Vaughan, T. B., 79, *162* (63); 95, 100, *162* (64)

Ventry, P., *168* (186)
Vinocur, R., 50, 112, 155, *160* (34)
Volavka, J., 25, 64, 69, 70, 86, 89, 95, 96, 103, 108, 119, 122, 135, 156, *161* (50); 43, 86, *161* (58); 21, 64, 67, 79, 80, 86, 95, 100, 108, 135, *168* (193); 79, 80, 86, 95, 99, 135, 136, *168* (194); 80, 95, *168* (195)
Vouyoucas, C. N., 9, *168* (196)

Walton, R. P., 39, *168* (197)
Wang, R. I., 69, 70, 145, *163* (84)
Waskow, I. E., 30, 70, 103, *168* (198)
Watanabe, A. M., 145, *168* (201)
Wechsler, D., 44, *168* (199)
Weil, A., 25, 37, 42, 63, 69, 70, 103, 110, 132, 135, 145, *168* (200)
Weingarten, H., 132, *167* (176)
Weingartner, H., 79, *162* (63); 95, 100, *162* (64)
Weiss, J. L., 145, *168* (201)
Wendkos, M. H., 157, *168* (202)
West, L. J., 38, 147, *165* (122)
Whitaker, C. A., 103, 110, *166* (161)
White, R., 70, *159* (9)

Wig, N. N., 154, *165* (123a)
Wikler, A., 121, 158, *168* (203); 157, 158, *168* (204); 25, 43, 79, 96, 103, 111, 121, 123, 135, 147, *169* (205)
Williams, E. G., 25, 43, 79, 96, 103, 111, 121, 123, 135, 147, *169* (205)
Williams, M. J., 43, 57, 60, *160* (26)
Williams, R. B., 108, *165* (136)
Wingfield, M., 25, 63, 119, 122, *166* (145)
Woo-Sam, J. M., 46, *169* (209)
Wootton, Lady, 156, *169* (206)
Wyatt, R. J., 79, *162* (63); 95, 100, *162* (64); 132, *167* (176)

Young, W. M., 154, 156, *169* (207)

Zabathas, E., *169* (208)
Zaks, A., 25, 64, 69, 70, 86, 89, 95, 96, 103, 108, 119, 122, 135, 156, *161* (50); 79, 80, 86, 95, 99, 135, 136, *168* (194)
Zimmerman, I. L., 46, *169* (209)
Zinberg, N. E., 25, 37, 42, 63, 69, 70, 103, 110, 132, 135, 145, *168* (200)